Breakthrough Women's Running

Dream Big and Train Smart

Neely Spence Gracey

Cindy Kuzma

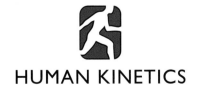

HUMAN KINETICS

Library of Congress Cataloging-in-Publication Data

Names: Gracey, Neely Spence, 1990- author. | Kuzma, Cindy author.
Title: Breakthrough women's running : dream big and train smart / Neely
   Spence Gracey, Cindy Kuzma.
Description: Champaign, IL : Human Kinetics, [2023] | Includes
   bibliographical references and index.
Identifiers: LCCN 2021051284 (print) | LCCN 2021051285 (ebook) | ISBN
   9781718206915 (paperback) | ISBN 9781718206922 (epub) | ISBN
   9781718206939 (pdf)
Subjects: LCSH: Running for women. | Running--Training. | Women
   runners--Nutrition.
Classification: LCC GV1061.18.W66 G73 2023 (print) | LCC GV1061.18.W66
   (ebook) | DDC 796.42082--dc23/eng/20211122
LC record available at https://lccn.loc.gov/2021051284
LC ebook record available at https://lccn.loc.gov/2021051285

ISBN: 978-1-7182-0691-5 (print)

Senior Acquisitions Editor: Michelle Earle; **Developmental Editor:** Anne Hall; **Managing Editor:** Miranda K. Baur; **Copyeditor:** Erin Cler; **Indexer:** Andrea J. Hepner; **Permissions Manager:** Martha Gullo; **Senior Graphic Designer:** Joe Buck; **Cover Designer:** Keri Evans; **Cover Design Specialist:** Susan Rothermel Allen; **Photograph (cover):** Tracy Ann Roeser / Tracy Ann Creative; **Photographs (interior):** © Human Kinetics, unless otherwise noted; **Photo Asset Manager:** Laura Fitch; **Photo Production Specialist:** Amy M. Rose; **Photo Production Manager:** Jason Allen; **Senior Art Manager:** Kelly Hendren; **Illustrations:** © Human Kinetics; **Printer:** Versa Press

We thank TAC, Tracy Ann Creative, in Boulder, Colorado, for assistance in providing the location for the photo shoot for this book.

Human Kinetics books are available at special discounts for bulk purchase. Special editions or book excerpts can also be created to specification. For details, contact the Special Sales Manager at Human Kinetics.

Printed in the United States of America

10 9 8 7 6 5 4 3 2 1

The paper in this book is certified under a sustainable forestry program.

Human Kinetics
1607 N. Market Street
Champaign, IL 61820
USA

United States and International
Website: **US.HumanKinetics.com**
Email: info@hkusa.com
Phone: 1-800-747-4457

Canada
Website: **Canada.HumanKinetics.com**
Email: info@hkcanada.com

E8336

Tell us what you think!
Human Kinetics would love to hear what we can do to improve the customer experience. Use this QR code to take our brief survey.

Breakthrough Women's Running

Dream Big and Train Smart

Contents

PART IV

Foreword

I believe movement is life. If you're not moving, you're dead, and I'm not ready to die yet. Running is something that has very much made me feel alive, giving me tools to conquer and overcome any sort of setback. It has brought me perspective, allowed me to appreciate the little things, and kept me excited about what's next.

I've always thrived on goals and challenges—short-term pursuits that are slightly intimidating, but still feel good, mentally and physically. You start at the beginning, there's an end to it, and then you're ready for the next one. No matter where you are in your fitness journey, you can be creative in using physical challenges to reach a goal and stay motivated.

Through my 15 years as a professional athlete, my primary goals were to make Olympic teams and U.S. teams, and I did. I won seven national championships between 2007 and 2015, and I finished fourth in the Olympic finals in the 800 meters in 2012.

I always knew having kids was something I also wanted to do, but it wasn't really talked about in the athletic world. I started thinking about it and cobbling together resources. I had the support of my coach, who had studied exercise physiology, and a great health care team. They knew staying active during pregnancy—in whatever way it was possible—would help me recover and return to high performance.

My goals looked a little different during those times. During the first trimester of my first pregnancy, I could only run-walk for about 20 minutes, but I always felt better when I did. My second trimester, I felt like a superhero, and I was able to get back to the track and the trails. By the end of my third trimester, with about four weeks left to go, I was tired more often than not, mostly from carrying the extra weight of the baby. I quickly found out that the energy I had for the day was the energy I had for the day, whether it was spent on good blood flow or existing in the same spot I woke up in. The difference? My mood vastly improved when I spent that energy on moving.

In 2014, I ran the U.S. track championships while eight months pregnant with my daughter, Linnea. I did the same thing in 2017, five months pregnant with my son, Lennox, wearing a Wonder Woman top and two flowers in my hair. The point of those performances was to show women there weren't any negative repercussions to movement. Also, running was my job. I believed I could do both—pursue my passion for running and have a family.

On the career side, I faced challenges, including a lack of support from my sponsors. I talked about this in a powerful *New York Times* op-ed in 2019, which launched the #DreamMaternity movement. So many women face pregnancy discrimination in the workplace and in sports. Those types of negative messages impact us physically and mentally, and I wanted to counteract them.

There's a lot women are told they can't do from the beginning. Add pregnancy to that, then motherhood. Misinformation continues to oppress and stifle us. Right now, we need more resources to answer women's questions, reassurances of what's possible, and voices inspiring us to continue to be our very best selves. That includes running, and it can include running within pregnancy.

That's why I'm so excited this book is here at this time. Neely and I have known each other through the professional running scene for years, and when she became a mother a few years after me, we connected on a different level. She has combined her experiences with research and input from experts into a guide to help women runners understand their bodies and minds in training at every phase of their lives; it's extremely necessary, and I'm encouraged to be a part of it.

I might not be aiming for Olympic teams right now, but as I continue my work as an athlete and activist, it's important for me to take on new challenges, including long-distance trail races and my first marathon, a stretch for someone who thrived running two laps of the track. Physical goals can change and be valuable as long as they're meaningful for you. Your goal might be to complete 26.2, come back to running pain-free postpartum, or reach that next athletic level. No matter where you're starting, you can challenge yourself to hit your peak performance. And *Breakthrough Women's Running* is an important tool in helping you get there.

Alysia Montaño
Olympian; seven-time national champion; three-time mom;
co-founder of nonprofit &Mother; Olympic sports analyst;
author of *Feel-Good Fitness* (VeloPress, 2020)

Preface

BUILDUP TO BOSTON MARATHON, APRIL 18, 2016

My mantra: "Attitude, believe, commit."

As I stood at the starting line in Hopkinton, prepared to make my marathon debut, I knew I was meant to be there. After all, my dad—Olympic marathoner Steve Spence—was running the race the day I was born. Exactly 50 years prior, Bobbi Gibb had become the first woman to complete this race. It felt like I was stepping into my destiny—my own place in history.

From the time I started in the sport in eighth grade, I'd been doing everything in my power to set big goals and run them down. By this point, I'd had my share of victories, including eight Division II NCAA Championships, a four-year pro career, and several first-place finishes at half marathons. Now I was taking the leap to the marathon. And not just any marathon—the Boston Marathon, the world's oldest, most storied 26.2-mile road race. When it comes to distance running, the stage doesn't get much bigger than that.

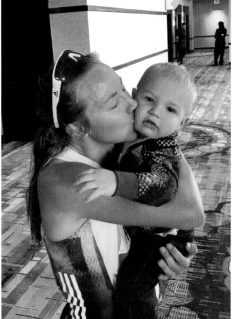
Neely Spence Gracey

Since the end of December 2015, I'd logged 1,325 miles specifically in preparation for this moment. On top of long runs and twice-weekly hard workouts, every hour of every day was precisely calibrated to set myself up for success. Every night, I turned my lights out by 9:00 p.m. I drove as far as two hours each way for massages, dry needling, and strength-training sessions. In four months, I went through three tubs of recovery protein, 10 pairs of shoes, and five bags of Epsom salts.

I'd hit a few bumps in the road, including a blister on one foot and a bone bruise on the other. I also carried the weight of high expectations. Some were my own, but there was undoubtedly a spotlight on me. Besides being the daughter of an Olympian, I faced high expectations because I'd forgone the Olympic Marathon Trials the prior February to make my debut at this prestigious event. Journalists, fans, and my competitors were watching me closely. I've always run with my whole heart, but this time, I felt like I had more to prove.

I put that all out of my mind as the race began. For the first few miles on the long, downhill slope through Ashland and into Framingham, the lead pack of women traveled at a relaxed pace. No one wanted to take the lead, and while I knew the marathon should feel easier than shorter distances at the start, I was anxious to find my groove. So at mile four, I stepped out to the front.

For the next two miles, I led the race, along with fellow American Sarah Crouch. We kept stealing glances at each other and smiling. I'd planned my whole life around this sport, but still, nothing can quite prepare you for the feeling of leading the Boston Marathon. We both knew it was a once-in-a-lifetime experience.

The leaders left us at around 10K, but Sarah and I stuck together. We'd run together, stride for stride, so many times over the years, competing against each other in Division II. Although we both aimed to be top American, we realized working as a team would bring the best out of each other. When I questioned myself near the halfway point, she encouraged me; when she hit a rough patch in the hills, I took my turn blocking the wind.

At Heartbreak Hill—around 20 miles—the time came for me to give my all. I pulled away from Sarah, my thoughts focused firmly on the finish line. I had a time goal in mind—2:35—and if I wanted to reach it, every step mattered. *Inhale. Exhale. Drive your knees. Hips forward. Relax your arms. Only 10K to go—you've run that so many times before.* I gradually picked up the pace. On my left, I passed train tracks and realized I was moving faster than the locomotive.

Finally, I made the famous last turn—right on Hereford, then left on Boylston, toward the finish line. The roar of the crowds was a force field pushing me forward. I poured every last ounce of strength and power into the final stretch. (Literally—this was the only time I've puked after a race!) Later, when I looked at my watch, I'd see I ran the final 400 meters in 71 seconds, a 4:46 mile pace.

I crossed the finish line in exactly 2 hours and 35 minutes, placing ninth overall and first American. When journalists appeared with microphones, I could barely speak. I thought of my dad running the same race, then proceeding to win a bronze medal at the World Championships and make an Olympic team. He's always inspired me, but now, I wholeheartedly believed I could follow in his footsteps. I'd conquered a new distance, catapulted my career forward, and opened my mind to new possibilities for my future—the very definition of a breakthrough.

BUILDUP TO HOUSTON MARATHON, 2020

My mantra: "Do what I can do with where I'm at right now and with the time that I have available."

Fast-forward to the winter of 2020. In some ways, my situation was similar—I was still living in Colorado with my husband and coach, Dillon; running professionally; and setting my sights on big goals. Specifically, I was hoping to qualify for the 2020 Olympic Marathon Trials.

But in other ways, life had been turned upside down. After a lingering foot injury led me to forgo running the New York City Marathon in 2017 as I'd planned, I decided to chase one of my other goals—becoming a mom. In July 2018, I gave birth to my son, Athens.

Though I had every intention of running through pregnancy, my body had other ideas. After childbirth, my comeback was hard, mentally and physically. Shifting hormone levels led to fatigue and injury, my anxiety levels were unlike anything I'd experienced, and sleep was a rare luxury.

I started back with a run-walk in September 2018 and then, after fracturing my femur, did the same thing again a year later. One day, I headed out for 10 minutes on the trail behind our Boulder home. My pace was slow, but my effort felt as if I were racing. When I turned around, I thought, *Could I make it back home?* I wasn't sure.

For someone whose life was defined by her athletic accomplishments, the uncertainty felt devastating. Seeing how unhappy I was, Dillon asked whether I was sure I wanted to keep racing. It took me a few weeks to answer him.

Somewhere inside, though, a small fire still flickered. I'd qualified for the Trials twice but never made it to the starting line. I couldn't yet let go of the possibility or fathom the thought of waiting four more years. Day by day, step by step, I moved forward.

I can clearly recall the first five-mile run that didn't feel terrible—it was early November 2019. By the end of the month, I decided I still wanted to try to qualify for the Trials. I set my sights on the Houston Marathon in January, which was the last day in the qualifying window.

My buildup looked radically different. I did one hard running workout a week instead of two, gave myself a day off each week when my body told me I needed it, and tried to sneak in naps when Athens did instead of cross-training or doing a second run. My instincts told me I could run the 2:45 qualifying time. But after two years away from racing, I was no longer sure I trusted them.

This race, I started not with the lead pack but with a pace group of 20-plus women, all targeting the goal of a Trials qualifier. There was the teamwork I'd felt with Sarah, amplified, as we shared drink bottles and words of encouragement. The middle miles felt tough, hard enough that I second-guessed myself, wondering whether I'd aimed too high. Still, I committed to giving it my all.

I broke away from the group after 22 miles, aiming to pick up my pace and finish strong. Unlike in Boston, my legs didn't respond with speed or springiness. So with around 3,000 meters to go, I tucked in behind another runner and did my best to hang on until the finish.

When I crossed the line in 2:44:03, securing my spot at the Olympic Trials in Atlanta at the end of February, I felt the same surge of pride and accomplishment. (I also felt gratitude—I gave a huge hug to my impromptu pacer as well as so many of the other women who ran OTQs.)

It was my slowest marathon—but my proudest one. For Boston and New York, I was trained, fit, and ready to perform at my peak. For this one, I was far less prepared, but I did it anyway. I'd overcome so much and proven I had a future in the sport. Even more than that, I realized I still wanted one. For as different as it looked, it was undoubtedly another breakthrough.

BUILD UP TO YOUR NEXT BIG GOAL, BEGINNING RIGHT NOW

Your mantra: "Trust the process."

The fact that these two stories can fill the same runner's training log demonstrates just how individualized the road map to a breakthrough can be.

Underlying each of these performances were consistent, solid strategies you can use to take your own running to the next level: Know the desired outcome but focus on the process. Turn off comparisons, both to others and to your own past. Create a plan that honors where you are now so you can become your best in the future.

Look, this running thing—it's not easy. I can tell you from experience, though, just how rewarding and fulfilling it can be. If you're picking up this book, you're probably aware of how the confidence and joy created by achieving your goals on the track or the roads carry over into the rest of your life. You're just looking for the right tools and information to get you there.

That's where we come in. With my experience as an elite distance runner and a coach who's guided over 500 runners through everything from their first 5K to an Olympic Trials qualifying time of their own, I know what it takes to craft a personalized plan for running success. And now I've teamed up with a longtime running journalist and

BREAKTHROUGH DEFINED

In sports media, the word *breakthrough* is often used to describe an athlete's first notable success—the time she won her first big collegiate title, emerged on the national scene, or appeared on the radar as a contender for Olympic squads and championship teams.

When we talk about a breakthrough, we mean a performance that breaks through a physical or mental barrier, taking your fitness and confidence to the next level. It's an accomplishment that lights you up when you think about it—and when you achieve it, or even surpass it, it changes your world.

While breakthroughs are often personal-best times, they aren't always. Your version might be as follows:

- A race that qualifies you for another competition, such as the Boston Marathon or the Olympic Trials
- The first time you complete or truly compete at a new distance
- Your first—or your fastest—race after a pregnancy, injury, or other extended break
- Any accomplishment that opens your mind to what's possible for you, convincing you to dream bigger

One interesting thing I've noticed in my career is that breakthroughs often come after periods of struggle. Every runner, if she keeps it up for a while, will eventually hit a rough patch—a time when she might plateau, fall short of her goals, or give it all on race day only to have a result that doesn't align with what she would have done in training. Those setbacks or challenges aren't fun, but they're often catalysts for the change and growth that ultimately propel her forward.

It makes sense when you think about it. Humans are often resistant to change, but if you keep doing the same things, you'll get the same results. It's in those moments of frustration that you feel motivated to reflect on everything from the goals you set in the first place to the steps you took along the way. You adjust and adapt and often end up even surprising yourself with what you can accomplish.

So if you're in the middle of one of those downturns—take heart. I believe better days are ahead of you. And if you're on an upswing right now, that's great! You can use the processes of goal setting and fine-tuning to take the next step—or leap—forward.

---

author to bring you a comprehensive guide to setting big goals, then building a system of daily habits and small steps to achieve them.

LEVELING UP

If you're like a lot of runners, you have big goals and a lot of ideas about how to reach them—sometimes too many! You've likely tried coaching yourself, looking at training ideas online, following pro runners and coaches on Instagram or Twitter, and watching videos on YouTube. You've had some success but just don't feel like everything's clicked for you.

You're ready for a little more guidance—a step-by-step guide on how to build not just a training plan but a lifestyle that supports your goals. You seek a mindset that moves you forward rather than holding you back. You want a system to overcome injuries, setbacks, and ebbs in motivation, incorporating the nuances of women's hormonal systems and pregnancy plans. You'd love simple, easy-to-implement options for cross-training, strength work, mobility, and core training. You need a strong base, a focused training block, and a plan to get from where you are to where you want to be, all with a strategic, progressive approach that builds confidence as well as fitness.

In short, you're looking for a plan that'll lead to your *Breakthrough*. We're so glad you've found it!

CALL ME YOUR COACH

From the earliest days of my running career, I've been soaking up as much knowledge as possible on how to run stronger, faster, and smarter. (It helps that this curiosity also runs in my genes—throughout his running career, my dad was always innovating.)

I graduated from Shippensburg University with a coaching minor and a major in communications studies. I strongly believe that effective coaching requires speaking (and writing) clearly, concisely, and effectively, and this education provided the foundation I needed to combine these pursuits.

I launched my business, Get Running Coaching, in 2013. Since then, I've helped hundreds of athletes accomplish their goals. Although I've worked with a wide range of runners, from elementary school students and high schoolers to older men aiming for personal records or Boston-qualifying times, my primary expertise and passion lie with coaching women near the prime of their running years. As a coach, I've seen and felt their struggles, weaknesses, doubts, and fears and watched them rise above it all, surprising even themselves.

What's most rewarding to me is when I see a breakthrough coming. I can often predict an outstanding performance before the athletes realize what's about to unfold. I see it in their training paces, sure, but also their emotional state—the way they've prepared diligently, responded quickly, and asked questions with curiosity and enthusiasm.

I make sure I tell them what I'm observing, as one last boost to their confidence. I know how much it has meant to me when coaches have shared their belief in my preparation and abilities, and I aspire to give that to my runners. I want them to know that when they toe the starting line, I'm just as nervous and excited as I am for my own races. For me, there's no greater victory than the phone call or text I get afterward—especially the ones that come with a triumphant finishing photo and a sense of awe in what they just accomplished.

Though we're just now meeting, I have good feelings about you too. You've clearly invested enough in the sport and yourself to pick up a book dedicated to making you better. I'm thrilled to offer you this compilation of what I've learned, observed, and experienced to guide you. I can already see the determination and focus you'll put into implementing the ideas in these pages and fine-tuning a plan that offers you exactly what *you* need to succeed. And I can tell you, you're on the verge of doing something truly special.

No one needs to give you the permission or the power to achieve your next big running goal—you already have what it takes to make it happen. By the time you finish this book, you'll understand exactly how to unlock your potential. As long as you're ready and willing to do the work—and have fun along the way—it's time for your next breakthrough.

Acknowledgments

FROM CINDY AND NEELY

We felt overwhelmed with inspiration after hearing the stories of our highlighted athletes. To Sara Hall, Tina Muir, Molly Huddle, Starla Garcia, Elise Cranny, Sara Vaughn, Nell Rojas, Emily Infeld, Mechelle Lewis Freeman, Amanda Nurse, Becky Wade, and Dr. Megan Roche: we are incredibly appreciative of your participation, and *Breakthrough* would not be the same without your contributions. Thank you also to the experts who helped fill our chapters with accurate and scientifically proven recommendations and information. Dr. Candice Zientek, Carrie Jackson, Dr. Shelby Harris, Dr. Stacy Sims, Celeste Goodson, Dr. Sara Tanza, Dr. Christine Abair, Christie Foster, Dr. Heather Linden, and again, Starla Garcia and Dr. Megan Roche, your knowledge and research were invaluable. Finally, this entire book would not have been possible without the ideas, support, and guidance of Human Kinetics, and especially Michelle Earle, Anne Hall, Martha Gullo, and Miranda Baur. Thank you for giving us a platform and opportunity, and for your editing expertise and positive feedback throughout the writing and editing process. We are also grateful to copyeditors Karla Walsh and Erin Cler for their assistance making the words shine, and senior graphic designer Joe Buck for bringing our creative vision to life on the page.

FROM NEELY

Writing a book has been on my bucket list since college, but without unwavering encouragement from you, Dillon, I don't know if I would have ever believed it could really happen. Hugs to my two little boys—both of you have brought so much perspective, joy, and love into my life. Thank you, Cindy, for being the most wonderful co-author and allowing me the chance to learn so much about the process while not feeling incredibly overwhelmed and lost.

Thank you to the whole team at Human Kinetics who rolled with my surprise pregnancy—Rome's arrival coincided with our original deadline, but so many people shifted schedules to make things happen. I envisioned colorful photos and the Colorado mountains, and, Tracy Roeser, you delivered with these gorgeous shots—I am so grateful. Lastly, thanks to my high school and college teammates, training partners over the years, mentors and coaches, friends, family, and all the members of Get Running Coaching, who have been an ongoing source of motivation and inspiration for me. Thank you for being on my team during this endeavor and always.

FROM CINDY

Thank you to Neely, for allowing me the honor of helping tell your story—it's a gift to work with a co-author who's both an expert and an incredible human, willing to lead through example and also learn as she goes. I'm so excited for your next chapter and your future breakthroughs! Thanks to all the editors who have given me the chance to write about these topics through the years, building a knowledge base and a list of sources to draw on (including, but not limited to, Sarah Lorge Butler, Brian Dalek, Christa Sgobba, Jen Ator, and Jessica Campbell-Salley). Huge gratitude to my parents Bill and Mary Szelag, my second parents Matt and Charlene Kuzma (and Lucas too), the coaches who have guided my own running, and all the friends I've shared miles and stories with through the years. And most of all, to Matt, for all the things. You're still the best decision I've made, and I don't know where I'd be without your support.

Introduction

YOUR ROAD MAP TO GREATNESS

In *Breakthrough*, we touch on just about everything you need to know to set yourself up for running success. We'll start in chapter 1 with goal setting, walking you through the process of selecting targets that are big enough to fuel you and realistic enough to ground you. Then we'll show you exactly how to break that big goal down into small, daily process goals that move you toward your destination.

That's truly the secret sauce, I've found, to turning lofty aspirations into real-life performances. Anyone can say they want to run faster, but actually turning that intention into results takes small, tangible changes to your everyday habits and routines. Over time, these build on themselves, propelling you ahead by leaps and bounds.

The chapters in this book will give you all the tools and advice you'll need to reach your goals:

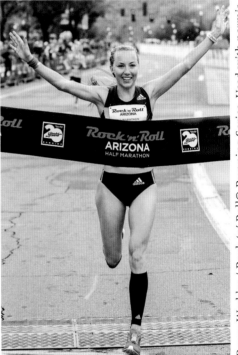

Bruce Wodder / Rock 'n' Roll® Running Series. Used with permission of World Triathlon Corporation.

- Training fundamentals and logistics, from choosing a plan to why (and how) to run by feel (chapter 2)

- Recovery, complete with two ways to track your physiology so you know you're striking the right balance between hard work and rest (chapter 3)

- Nutrition basics, including five recipes directly from my kitchen to yours, to fuel your training (chapter 4)

- The latest science on how your menstrual cycle affects your performance and how to work with your hormones to improve your training and racing (chapter 5)

- Pregnancy and postpartum running, a particular passion of mine (chapter 6)

- Exactly how—and why—to build strength and cross-training into your schedule, along with four resistance routines you can do with minimal equipment (chapter 7)

- Why "listening to your body" isn't enough, and more on the nitty gritty of injury prevention; also, 20 different mobility moves to target your problem areas (chapter 8)

- Mantras, mindfulness, and more ways mindset work is critical to pair with your physical training (chapter 9)

- The incredible power of breathing and the counting trick that's led me to my own breakthroughs (chapter 10)

At the end of each chapter, you'll find a section called From Barrier to Breakthrough. There, we'll provide a ready-made selection of small, tangible actions—we call them breakthrough goals—geared to the specific obstacle you need to overcome.

Know you *should* strength train but just can't figure out when to squeeze it into your schedule? Check page 107 for three secrets to success. Constantly fading at the end of a hard workout? See page 136 for three techniques to help you stay strong. There's also help for coping with injury (page 124), how to work with your body during pregnancy and what to do if you can't run at all (page 87), and stocking your kitchen so you'll always have the perfect postrun snack (page 42).

In chapters 12 through 15, you'll find a full array of training plans for distances from 5K to marathon as well as a beginner or return-to-running program for after injury or pregnancy. In chapter 16, we'll talk more about setbacks and how to navigate through them. Finally, in chapter 17, on page 201, you'll find a template and guide to putting all these pieces together—including those breakthrough goals—into one solid, personalized plan.

All the advice in *Breakthrough* is grounded in science and evidence as well as stories from my own personal experience as an elite runner and coach. (You'd better believe there are a few choice nuggets from my 17-plus years of handwritten logs.) You'll also ready content directly from experts in training, physiology, and psychology as well as other inspiring female athletes who share the secrets behind their own breakthroughs.

HOW TO USE THIS BOOK

For starters, we'd recommend reading it through from start to finish to gain an overview of all the components that go into a breakthrough. Keep some sticky notes or a notepad handy. As you read through, notice the tips and goals that excite you and flag them. If you feel inspired, you can put down the book and try something on the spot, for instance, a breathing exercise (page 140) or side-lying quad stretch (page 119).

Once you've read through the book, we recommend going back to the chapters that were most eye-opening for you, spoke to your specific situation, or offered solutions to obstacles you're currently facing.

Next, head to the From Barrier to Breakthrough section at the end and pick one to three process goals to work on at a time. The more specific you can be, the better. For instance, rather than "focus on hydration," your process goal could be "drink 90 ounces a day."

Now, flip to chapter 17—Get It Together, on page 199—to see how to plug those process goals into your bigger training plan (you can even download a tracker on my website at https://getrunningcoaching.com/breakthrough). That way, you can seamlessly integrate them into your training.

Finally, keep the book as a reference. Every month—or whichever interval you choose to check in on your process goals—you can reevaluate how you did. When you've successfully built new habits, you can check back for ideas of other elements of your life you can fine-tune. And once you achieve your next big breakthrough, you can pull it back out and start plotting the next one.

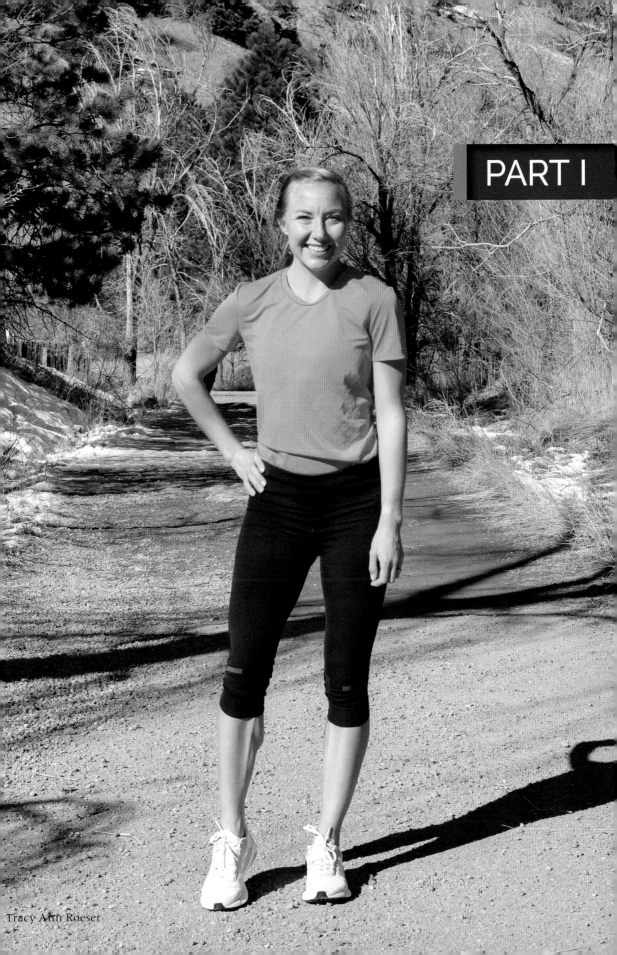

PART I

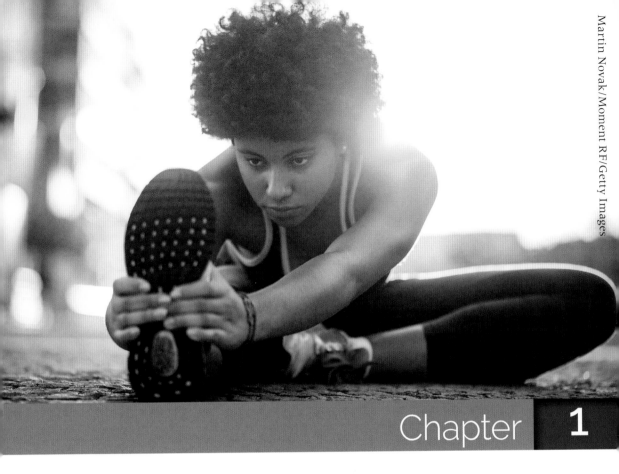

Chapter 1

Dream Big; Start Small

" 2020 gave us some high highs and low lows. Through it all, I hope I showed my kids how to never settle for playing it safe after disappointments, but to keep taking risks and putting yourself out there. Your breakthroughs may be just around the corner. "

Sara Hall, pro marathoner, American half-marathon record holder, and mother of four

A successful running journey begins with clear, compelling goals. That seems simple enough, but there's an art to setting goals that are right for you as an individual—they must be big enough to excite you but not so out of reach that they set you up for disappointment. They also need to acknowledge where you are right now in your running life and your life overall.

Do you already have a goal in mind? How clear and concrete is it? Is this your first time going after something bold and ambitious? Are you new to the process of structuring your training around one big target?

No matter what your experience level is with goals or how firmly you've settled on yours, you'll find ideas and guidance in this chapter. You'll need to consider factors such as your experience level and how much time you have to train and recover as well as the types of achievements that inspire and excite you. Start here to create short- and long-term outcome goals that motivate you, then break them down into process goals that get you from point A to point B with joy and confidence.

FROM VISION TO ACTION

Most runners would describe themselves as goal oriented. I'm no exception—one of my earliest goals was keeping up with my Olympic marathoner dad and lifelong runner mom. During our summers training at altitude, they'd take off on the Boulder Creek Path, my mom pushing my twin sisters in the double stroller. I couldn't keep up on foot, so I learned to bike at the age of three so I wouldn't be left behind!

By the time I started college at Shippensburg University, I knew the big things I wanted out of life: to be a coach, a wife, a mom, and a pro runner. Of course, wanting and doing are two different things. Visions of wedding dresses and shoe contracts provided powerful motivation, but making my dreams come true was up to me.

As stepping-stones to these bigger ambitions, I set interim goals. Some came from what felt personally exciting and rewarding, such as winning NCAA titles and representing the United States at international championships. Others focused on scoring points for the team at meets. Each season, I set specific time goals, aiming to PR at various distances.

Throughout, I talked to my dad, who was also my college coach, about what he thought was possible for me. As my career progressed, I sought inspiration and advice from an ever-expanding circle. Once Dillon and I started dating my freshman year, our shared fandom of the sport of running led to even more motivating discussions about my future. Each summer, when we traveled to Colorado for altitude training, I'd pepper the pros with questions about their progression.

The final piece of the puzzle came my sophomore year when I met sport psychology professor Dr. Candice Zientek. (You'll hear a lot more about her in chapter 9, on page 126.) From her, I learned to set not only outcome goals—achievements such as finishing times, placements, and national titles—but also process goals, the actual steps I'd take to achieve them.

In other words, aspiring to represent the United States in international competitions wasn't enough. I needed to define the training and racing strategies that would get me there and then plot specific ways to obtain them. With her help, broad proclamations turned into weekly and monthly goals and then daily actions.

For example, I often felt uncomfortable in a pack of runners. However, if I wanted to compete with the best, I wasn't always going to be in the lead; I had to learn to follow. To practice, I asked a speedy teammate whether I could run on her shoulder or directly behind her in track workouts. She agreed, and I grew more comfortable in those positions with each speed session. I knew that I could follow and then set up a strong kick to win when I got into the right race.

In the spring of 2011, my junior year of college, I lined up with some of the country's best athletes in the 5K at the prestigious Mt. SAC Relays in California. Competing against Sara Hall, Jenny Simpson, and Molly Huddle (she held the American record for the 5K at that time), I used the techniques I'd built in those weekly speed sessions to finish 10th. My 15:33:83 was not only a 34-second personal best (then a breakthrough for me), but it was also the fastest 5K time in NCAA Division II history.

This performance, on the day before my 21st birthday, catapulted my confidence to the next level. I could—and I *did*—compete with some of the nation's best. Those big dreams of running professionally were now starting to seem more tangible and achievable. After graduating, I started my pro career by signing with a team called the Hansons Brooks Original Distance Project.

Using the same principle of picturing the outcome while focusing on the day-to-day steps required to reach it also worked in other parts of my life. The details of goal setting in your career, relationships, and family are probably best addressed by coaches in those fields rather than here on these pages. But I know I'm not the only runner who's found that success in one area can provide a blueprint for how to achieve in any area.

I still have yet to realize two big dreams for my pro running career—a sub-2:30 marathon and a national title. I ran my 2:34:55 marathon PR on the notoriously tough New York City course, but I bonked near the end. However, I feel confident I could run five minutes faster with proper training, a fast course, and a better fueling strategy. As for the title, well, I've come in second seven times, so first seems well within my capabilities if things go right on race day.

In other words, they're just the type of stretches that, if I reach my hand out far enough, I believe I can touch. Every day, week, month, and year, I lay out the specifics of how I intend to reach those goals. Of course, the outcome isn't always exactly what I'd anticipated; for instance, I didn't exactly plan my second pregnancy, though now I can't imagine life without Rome! But with this road map in mind, I can adjust, adapt, and continue striving, no matter what life throws at me.

TRANSCEND YOUR LIMITS

Working as a running coach has given me a front-row seat into athletes' biggest dreams and desires. I get so excited about that first email, phone call, or meeting when a runner lays it all on the line.

Some want to qualify for the Boston Marathon or Olympic Marathon Trials. Others seek a personal best time, or to conquer a new distance, or to reintegrate running into their lives as mothers. In short, they're looking to make a breakthrough of their own, and they're asking for my help. What an honor!

I know that to open up about your audacious goals takes guts. I'm beyond grateful when athletes share, and from the moment we agree to work together, I feel invested in bringing their visions to life.

We all need big goals to fuel our efforts. Most of us are capable of far more than we think, provided we give ourselves the time and tools we need to succeed (much more on all that in chapter 2, page 13).

So if you're a runner with a goal that lights you up, gets you out of bed in the morning, and makes you equal parts scared and excited, you're in the right place. I get it; I'm thrilled for you, and I'm willing to work with you to make it happen.

Don't stress, though, if you're still figuring it all out. I also work with plenty of runners who know they want more out of themselves but aren't quite sure where to focus. If you don't yet have a concrete goal, here are some things you might think about to spark ideas:

- *Consider how close you are to meeting a specific qualifying time.* Some common goals include the Boston Marathon; Olympic Marathon Trials; or automatic entry into other major marathons, such as Berlin, Chicago, or New York City.

- *Recall the race distances you've competed at before.* Is there one at which you think you can get faster or a new distance you haven't tried but would like to? (Note: This doesn't always have to be a longer race. I know plenty of marathoners who get thrills from training for a fast mile or 5K.)

- *Talk to other runners you know.* If you have regular training partners, they might have goals that resonate with you too. Or if you know runners a little ahead of you in pace or experience level, ask about an accomplishment that was particularly meaningful for them.

- If you're scrolling on social media and you feel a pang of jealousy at seeing someone else's medal pic or finish-line victory pose, take notice. That likely means you're drawn toward a similar goal. (Note: This is probably the only time I'd suggest comparing yourself to others on social media.)

- Ponder longer-term ambitions, such as earning your Six Star Finisher Medal by running all the World Marathon Majors, running a half or full marathon in every state, or maintaining a streak at a specific event.

NEXT, GET REAL

Often, immediately after runners share a big goal, they seek validation. *This is what I'm aiming for,* they'll say. *Do you think I can do it?*

You might have a similar question on your mind as you plan for your own breakthrough. I understand that too. While big dreams inspire me, I'm the type of runner who also wants targets that are realistic—things I know that I have a reasonably good chance of achieving if I work hard.

Of course, I don't have a crystal ball. Sure, I can use tools such as pacing charts and race prediction calculators, but I don't have a simple, scientific algorithm into which I can plug your current stats and guarantee specific results. Your performance (and mine) is determined by infinite factors from genes to consistency in training to the weather on race day.

But there are patterns among the athletes who turn their dreams into reality. Here are the factors I'd encourage you to consider when evaluating a goal.

How Far You Have to Go

If you're a five-hour marathoner aiming to finish in less than three hours, you have a bigger gap to cover than someone who's run 3:35 and needs to beat 3:30 to qualify for Boston or someone who's run a half marathon in 1:35. That doesn't mean it's not possible! However, you might need to allow extra time or make more dramatic shifts to your routine.

How Long You Have to Get There

We sometimes decide big goals aren't possible when, in fact, the problem lies in how quickly we're aiming to achieve them. With some exceptions (which we'll talk about shortly), runners rarely take 100 steps forward at a time. And even if you do set a massive personal best in one race, you're likely to make more incremental progress the next time.

Knowing and planning for this can keep you from feeling discouraged. If you can set aside a substantial amount of time to target your breakthrough—perhaps a year, with multiple blocks of training within it—you're far more likely to get there as well as to have fun along the way. I had a runner come to me recently who was planning three years ahead—my dream client!

What You've Done Before

Many new runners go through a period when, as their bodies adapt to the sport, they become faster with every race. Eventually, though, you'll probably reach a plateau. It's a bit of a cruel twist, but the more experience and years of training you have, the harder fought the victories.

Every once in a while, I'll see even experienced runners make a huge leap forward—say, taking 30 minutes off their marathon time—by filling an obvious gap in training. For instance, runners who have prepared for marathons with only easy running can see swift progress when they begin speedwork (we'll talk about that in chapter 2, page 17), and in half and full marathons, fueling properly during the race can make a huge difference (all about this in chapter 4, page 37). But these huge leaps aren't typical, nor do they usually happen multiple times for the same runner.

How Open You Are to Change

Similarly, if you want a result you've never seen, you'll have to alter something about your training to make it happen. Some people start with training consistently over a long time, not just in the days and weeks before a race. The bigger your base of mileage, the stronger the foundation you have to build on. If you run consistently for six months to a year before starting an official 20-week marathon training plan, you'll likely see better results than if you started that same plan after a long break.

But if you've been reliably putting in the work and progress just isn't coming, you'll have to shake up something else. This might mean adding in more or different kinds of workouts, building in more recovery time (all about that in chapter 3, page 27), taking a training cycle to focus on the 5K (there's a plan for that on page 161) before trying another marathon, prioritizing strength training (see page 177), or racing more—or less—frequently.

Your Available Time and Energy

We'll talk more about how life stress affects your running—and what to do about it—in chapter 9, on page 128. While there are ways to reduce its effect, there are some instances when big goals just aren't compatible with the phase you're at in your life. For instance, if you have a new baby, are studying for a big test, have demanding work projects, or must provide care for a sick family member, you might find that too many long runs or hard workouts deplete you or you lack the time or resources to recover properly.

Being realistic doesn't mean giving up on your dreams. In fact, if you can simply get in some easy miles during these trying periods, you may build a stronger base that leaves you in the perfect position to aim higher than ever when circumstances change.

How Much Joy the Goal Brings You

Sometimes, runners set a certain goal because they think they "should" or they believe it represents the next logical step for them. But if your heart's not truly in it, you're going to have a much harder time sticking with things when the going gets tough.

As Brad Stulberg, a performance coach and cofounder of The Growth Equation, told *Time* magazine, "Before you take on a goal, visualize the process and how it makes you feel. If you become tight and constricted, it's probably not the right goal or time. If you feel open and curious, that's a good sign" (Loudin 2021).

Check in with yourself honestly. Just because you've run a few marathons doesn't mean you have to target a Boston qualifier (BQ) or Olympic Trials qualifier (OTQ) right now, or ever, if you don't want to. Running a fast 5K, or trying the mile, or seeing how long you can keep a consistent schedule in the midst of a busy life just might sound more exciting and fun. Find what truly ignites you, from the inside out, at this moment in time.

Whether You Can Authentically Celebrate Milestones Along the Way

Big goals provide strong motivation. But just like you need a gel or a sports drink to make it through a marathon, you require infusions of encouragement en route to reaching them—especially if, as I suggested before, you're committing to them for a longer time.

If you're aiming to go from a five-hour marathon to a sub-3:30 BQ, you might set goals of 4:30, 4:00, 3:45, and so on, knowing you're likely to make smaller amounts of progress the closer you get to your goal. The more you allow yourself to appreciate each step along the way, the easier it can feel to stay disciplined for the long haul.

Add It All Up: You've Got This!

The bottom line? In my experience, the runners who are most likely to achieve big goals allow themselves plenty of time to improve. They're willing to try new things, whether they be track workouts, deadlifts, or extra recovery days, and they celebrate every step along the way.

EVOLUTION OF A GOAL

Of course, to plan how you're going to get there, you need an idea of where you're going. When I'm planning a season, I set an outcome goal (time, placement, or both) at the beginning of a training cycle. That helps me determine everything, from where and when to race to the exact date I need to start training.

I always suggest that my runners set three outcome goals for each race—A, B, and C goals. I describe them this way:

A. Your stretch goal—your personal-best qualifying time or what you think you can push yourself to achieve if everything goes right

B. A slightly less ambitious, reasonably attainable goal if you have a decent race day

C. Your fallback goal—what you can feel satisfied with accomplishing even if the weather is terrible on race day or you miss some training because of injury (Finishing strong—or finishing, period—is often a great C goal, especially for longer distances.)

One of the beautiful things about training is that you can't always be sure what you're capable of until you start trying. Some athletes might find they're exceeding expectations and can race at an even faster pace than they'd planned. Others, meanwhile, might have an unexpected setback or realize they need a little more time for their bodies to adapt before they can reach their biggest dreams. (Note that accepting this fact doesn't make you a failure—it actually suggests you're a smart, dedicated athlete willing to maximize your potential.)

So midway through your training cycle, it's a good idea to take stock of these goals again. Your training paces—and any dress-rehearsal races you do (more about this on page 200)—can give you a solid idea of where you stand. If you're confidently running at or near your race pace in workouts during your biggest training block, you're probably on the right track. You can also consult the VDOT (short for $\dot{V}O_2$max) chart on page 156 in chapter 11 or an online race prediction calculator to help you clarify.

FIND YOUR DRIVE

Most successful runners have both big dreams and small goals along the way. But everyone has a slightly different motivational style, a way of deciding where to focus most that works best for their individual psychology.

Some runners thrive by putting lofty aims out there for the world to see. In November 2017, Gwen Jorgensen—already an Olympic gold medalist in the triathlon—announced she was transitioning to running full time, with a goal of winning Olympic gold in the marathon. It was a bold declaration; no American woman had won since Joan Benoit Samuelson prevailed in the first women's Olympic Marathon in 1984.

Jorgensen wound up skipping the 2020 Olympic Marathon Trials to focus on the track instead. As she told *Sports Illustrated* at the time, "My goals in the marathon aren't changing. My timeline is" (Chavez 2019). In March 2021, she improved her personal-best 5K time to 15:08:28, en route to the Olympic Track & Field Trials on the track that year. Even if she never wins another medal, who's to say she hasn't accomplished more than she would have if she hadn't put it all out there?

Marathoner Sara Hall (she's profiled on page 11) also focuses on her big dreams, even if she's a bit less public about the ways she expresses them. In 2020, she wrote "Olympic Marathon Trials Champion" on her bathroom mirror. When that didn't happen, she wrote instead, "American record-holder" and went for that at the Marathon Project in December (Crouse 2020). She fell short by just shy of a minute. She ran 2:20:32, compared to Deena Kastor's record of 2:19:36. And in January of 2022, she finally made her dream come true at the Aramco Houston Half Marathon, running 67:15 to break Molly Huddle's American record of 67:25.

Meanwhile, I'm the type of runner who knows her long-term goals and has them written in a journal. I'm not opposed to sharing them, but they're things that, based on the types of factors I previously listed, I feel nearly certain I can accomplish. And I spend a lot more time focusing on the next step in the process than the bigger dream, for instance, qualifying for the Olympic Marathon Trials before envisioning the Olympics themselves.

I used to wonder whether that meant I wasn't ambitious enough to succeed as a pro athlete, but now I know that it's just a difference in motivational style. I'm a planner who revels in the victory just around the corner; I find myself more excited about putting in the work for a goal that's right at my fingertips. If I spend a lot of time dwelling on faraway dreams that seem out of reach, I'll feel overwhelmed and defeated before I even begin.

As you plan for your own breakthrough, consider your personal tendencies and act accordingly. Does a vision board with your wildest dreams, a public declaration of bold ambition, or a daily reminder of what you hope for energize you? Use them if so; shout your goal from the rooftops (or, at least, on Instagram and Strava), scrawl it on your mirror, or make it the background on your phone. But if constant reminders leave you feeling more anxious about failure than eager to try harder, it's OK to hold your goals more closely and turn your mind instead to the next step of the journey.

Either way, congratulate yourself for figuring out what makes you tick. Runners who know themselves and leverage their strengths while working to improve their weaknesses are bound to go far.

Finally, I revisit my outcome goals one last time at the end of my training cycle—usually during the taper phase. At that point, I've put in all the hard work and have more than enough data to tell whether my A goal is still where I prefer it—a little bit scary but also exciting and motivating. I also make sure I can still sleep well at night if I achieve my B or C goal. If anything seems either too out of reach or not ambitious enough, I can adjust it.

This final check gives me a realistic expectation of what I can accomplish. And as a bonus, while I look back on all the workouts and races I've conquered, I feel even more ready to get out there and make it happen.

PLAN THE PROCESS

Up to this point, we've spent a lot of time discussing outcome goals, such as times, places, and qualifiers. Those are critical for success, but they can't stand alone. The key—what Dr. Zientek taught me years ago and many runners neglect—is to pair them with process goals. Again, these are the small steps you'll take every day to bring those big dreams to life, such as the speed workouts where I practiced following my teammate.

When I'm preparing for a big event, I usually set the outcome goals first and then work backward. For instance, for the 2016 Boston Marathon, I started focused training in December with the goal of a strong debut. By the end of January, I'd set solid outcome goals:

1. Run 2:35 or faster
2. Place in the top 10
3. Finish first among Americans

These were my A goals; each one also had a B and a C goal associated with it (for instance, as far as placement goes, top 15 was my B goal, and top 20 was my C goal).

But how, exactly, would I get there? I set these process goals:

1. *Learn how to fuel every 5K.* This meant practicing regularly on long runs with Osmo—the drink I had in my bottles—stationed every 5K along the course. Sometimes, Dillon would bring me bottles by bike or car; other days, I'd run short loops, passing a bottle stop every 30 minutes. I even did some runs with lemon-lime Gatorade, the fluid that was on the course in Boston, so I'd know I could use it if I happened to miss one of my prepared bottles.

2. *Get more comfortable at longer distances, for both workouts and long runs.* At this point, I'd spent most of my career focusing on the 5K and 10K—I'd done only three half marathons when I set my sights on Boston. I extended my long runs from a maximum of 18 miles to as long as 21 miles. As for workouts, I went from six-mile tempo runs to two by six-mile tempo runs—the first one at 6:06 pace and the second at 5:51—with one mile of easy running in between. Along the way, I practiced both my fueling and my mindset.

3. *Lock into a routine.* Starting about three weeks before Boston—when I hit my peak mileage—I wrote this phrase in big, bold letters in my training log: "Do less; focus more." (I even made it the screen saver on my phone.) I dialed in every last detail, from adding daily pool sessions to aid recovery to drinking enough water to refill my bottle by noon each day.

The phrase "trust the process" has long been one of my mantras (more on those on page 133). My Boston preparation brought this saying to life. Nailing all three of my process goals left me confident I'd prepared as well as I could for the race, and confidence is a powerful performance enhancer. (After that two by six-mile tempo, for instance, I wrote in my log, "I conquered.") That was less than three weeks out from race day, and when I revisited my outcome goals at that point, I realized they were exactly on point—challenging but possible.

That warm April day, I was able to achieve all three of my outcome goals—I ran 2:35:00 for ninth place overall and top American. Of course, things don't always play out so perfectly. But I firmly believe the reason they did is the combination of big goals and the little things I did consistently, time and again, to make them happen.

While I pride myself on providing smart, effective training plans to the runners I coach, I think it's my guidance on setting process goals that's perhaps the most valuable part of the equation. That's exactly why each chapter of this book ends with breakthrough goals—examples of small daily steps you can take that will help you bust barriers and take your running to the next level. Your list of process goals might not be as extensive or intense as the ones I made before Boston (even mine aren't always that focused or intense; that was a huge race for me!). But it's still important to have them outlined.

Once you've set your big outcome goals, work backward on smaller interim goals, then really drill down into the processes that will get you there. Revisiting your goals throughout the cycle will bring you the confidence you need to make it all come together. As you keep reading, you'll understand how to put the pieces together, including a template in chapter 17 to integrate these steps into your training and your life. It's in this delicate equilibrium—a balancing act between shooting for the moon and keeping your feet on the ground and moving forward—that true breakthroughs are born.

Embracing the Process: Sara Hall

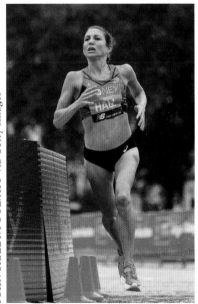

JOHN SIBLEY/POOL/AFP via Getty Images

Though she'd go on to many more accomplishments in her pro career, Sara Hall sees a high school race back in 2000 as her biggest breakthrough.

The one thing she'd wanted her whole career at Montgomery High School in Santa Rosa, California, was to win the Foot Locker Cross Country Championships. She placed third as a sophomore, failed to qualify as a junior, and started her senior year "in the worst shape of my high school career," she says.

Still, she didn't give up: "I visualized it every day my senior year as I did strides on a grass strip, envisioning winning in a sprint finish. Even though I lost many races that season, the biggest one ended up playing out just as I had rehearsed over and over."

Sara isn't afraid to follow her heart. She pursues the goals that light her on fire, writing them not just on her mirror but also in her training log and on notes that she reads the day before big races. It's hard for a runner to know whether all those big dreams are attainable, she admits. "But in the process, you get to find your potential."

FROM BARRIER TO BREAKTHROUGH

Chances are that you have goals in mind already, or you probably wouldn't be reading a book about reaching them. The chapters to come are full of small process goals to get you there, but here are a few that can help you start out on the right foot.

Barrier

I have a big goal in mind but have no idea where to start.

Breakthrough Goals

Choose one or more.

I will do the following:

- Reread this chapter, writing down my big goals and then thinking through the factors to consider
- Commit to reading this book to the end, flagging the parts that seem most relevant to my goals and situation along the way
- Work backward from my big goal to set a smaller goal for the next training block and then three process goals to achieve it

---

Barrier

I've never aimed this high before, and I'm not sure it's possible for me.

Breakthrough Goals

Choose one or more.

I will do the following:

- Calculate how far off I am right now
- Determine how long I'm willing to dedicate to achieving it
- Honestly evaluate my life right now and whether it's the right time to try for it

---

Barrier

I've tried for the same goal for years and keep falling short.

Breakthrough Goals

Choose one or more.

I will do the following:

- As I read through this book, note things that are very different from the way I currently train and live and choose one to three areas to focus on changing for the next training block
- For the next week, pay attention to how I respond when thinking about my goal so I can better understand my motivational style and adjust my focus as needed
- Identify a smaller, interim goal; set a realistic timeline for it; and choose a way to celebrate it

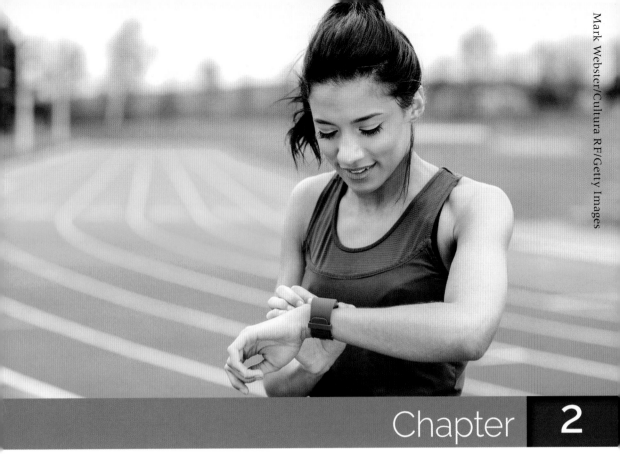

Mark Webster/Cultura RF/Getty Images

Chapter | 2

Plan Smart

"
There will be seasons in running where we are motivated and ready to get after it, but our life will not allow it to be the focus. There will be seasons when we do have the time, but motivation isn't there. And then there will be the seasons where they both align. Maybe not to have the perfect setup—life is always going to throw curveballs—but there is enough space, energy, time, and heart to go for it.
"

Tina Muir, host of the *Running for Real* podcast and author of *Overcoming Amenorrhea*

You've set your goals; now, it's time to build the foundation for reaching them. You have some decisions to make as you plan your training: Will you hire a coach, use a plan from this book, or find another option? Will you run alone or with a group, when and where will you run, and how will you track the results?

While there are some broad principles underlying success in distance running—such as building up your long run and progressing over time—many of these choices come down to understanding your unique psychology, physiology, and lifestyle. Take the time now to think through the logistics, factors as significant as where you live and train and as small as the watch you wear on your wrist. Then you can take steps to set yourself up for success—striving for your goal while having fun along the way.

FINDING MY FOOTING

Though pro running had long been a dream of mine, I can't say the transition into it was an easy one. I passed up my final track season of collegiate eligibility to sign with an agent and join the Hansons Brooks Original Distance Project, a professional running team based in suburban Detroit. The coaches—Keith and Kevin Hanson—taught me so much, and I remain grateful for the opportunity.

But from the beginning, it wasn't a good fit. I'd grown up in a small town, where most people knew me and those who didn't were outgoing and friendly. I was home-schooled but ran for the high school team, which offered a blend of independence and support in which I thrived. College—in the same town where my dad was the cross country coach—was no different.

In Michigan, I knew few other people than the team. The runners who had been there longer had families, social networks, and entire established lives. We all got along but didn't spend time together outside of practice. Although Dillon and I were already married, he was living far away from me in Houston. In the hours between practice and the gym, I often sat alone in my apartment above a shoe store. There were definitely kind and supportive people—including three families whom I keep in touch with to this day—and that helped me feel less lonely. Still, I felt myself sinking into sadness. When running and life got hard—as they inevitably did—I crumbled, shutting down instead of reaching out.

Everything changed in 2015 when I did an altitude stint in Boulder. Training on trails in the shadow of the mountains, I fell in love all over again—with the place, with running, with the belief I once had in myself and my abilities. Miraculously, at around the same time, Dillon got a job offer in Denver. In that moment, I knew I couldn't go back.

I quit the team, Dillon accepted the offer, and together we began building a life for the first time despite having been married for over two years. I recreated the entire support system I needed to run well—friends to train with, a strength coach to help build me up, a chiropractor and a physical therapist to address my aches and pains. It took time and hard work, but in a place I loved with a person I adored, I had the bandwidth to handle it.

When I look back on it now, I can see a lot I would have done differently. Right out of college, changing my mindset to focus on the positive and being more proactive about making connections would have absolutely improved my situation in Michigan. But ultimately, I don't think I ever would have run my best there. The more I learned about myself, the better I understood the essential elements of my happiness—what I truly needed to live well and therefore run well.

As you embark on your own big goal, I encourage you to spend some time thinking through what makes you tick, both as a runner and a person. There are a few basic non-negotiables for running your best, for instance, training in phases that build over time (see page 23) with ample recovery, all of which we'll talk about in a second—as well as some other strategies I strongly advocate for all my athletes (keeping a training log, for one, which we'll get into shortly). But so much of the rest is open to individualization.

For example, take the 2020 Olympic Marathon Trials. Not only did I qualify, but so did my college teammate Katie Spratford. Together, she and I coached three other women who qualified and competed under our guidance. One was a single 20-something with the ability to invest lots of time for training and recovery, one worked as a labor and delivery nurse with 12-hour shifts but frequent days off, and one was a wildlife biologist who spends late nights out researching owls. Each of us had a very different approach to training and racing, but it led us all—including me—to achieving that huge goal of an OTQ, then competing in Atlanta in 2020.

KNOW YOURSELF

Aligning your training and your life to point in the same direction—toward your goals—starts with self-reflection. The better you understand what has worked for you in the past and the realities of your present, the easier it is to make choices that support your desired future. Once you've firmly committed to your goals, take some dedicated time to sit down and consider your physiology, preferences, and the practicalities of your life.

Even if you've been running for years, it's extremely valuable to revisit not just your goals but also the way you'll plan to execute them at the beginning of a new year or training cycle. Think of it like the preseason planning you'd do with a coach (and if you decide to work with one, you'll have a jump-start on the process).

If you've kept training logs in the past, haul them out now. You might think you remember everything, but as I can tell you from working on this book, there are memories that won't come to the surface until prompted by something you've written. Also, have resources handy, such as your personal, family, work, and school calendars, and information about your goal race if you've already signed up for it.

Here are some questions to consider. Once you start planning, you might come up with a few more that are important to you.

- How much mileage can I comfortably handle? (Looking at what you've done in the past and how it relates to your injury history and race performances can help you figure this out.)
- Have I been injured frequently in the past? If so, can I pinpoint common underlying factors—and what I need to do to address them? (There's lots more on this in chapter 8, page 109.)
- How much of a base do I have right now? (In other words, how many weeks and months have you been running consistently, and what's your average weekly mileage?)
- How much time do I have to train—both in hours per day and days per week?
- When in the day will I do most of my running? And is my schedule fairly consistent, day to day, or does it vary a lot?
- Do I want to train alone, with one or two other people, or a larger group? And if I do want training partners, do I know how to find them?
- Who else in my life needs to be aware of my goals and habits? (We'll get into this more in Build Your Team, page 19.)

- Are there other family, personal, or life events I need to work around when planning my training?
- Can I get help with other responsibilities or take alternate steps to offload some stress? (There's more on this later.)
- Where will I run most of my mileage? Do I have a safe and appropriate place to do long runs as well as hills and track workouts at the times I need to do them? (We'll talk a bit more about some options in chapter 11, on page 151.)
- What other tools, gear, and gadgets do I want to consider acquiring? (See Gear Up, page 19.)
- When I look at the races, individual training sessions, and training cycles that left me feeling the most confident and joyful, what did they have in common?
- Similarly, can I identify any common factors behind races, workouts, or training cycles where I struggled the most?

USE YOUR STRENGTHS

The last two questions on that list offer insight into something I think is underappreciated in training. I would also recommend experienced runners ask themselves one slightly more specific version: Which type of runs do I enjoy the most and feel like I'm "best" at?

For instance, do you thrive on short, fast repetitions at the track, or do you prefer longer intervals, such as mile repeats? Do your training partners know you as the runner who crushes the downhills or the one who always has enough left in the tank to finish a long run strong? This tells you a lot about your strengths and weaknesses as a runner—incredibly valuable information if you know how to use it.

The trick? Do more of what you're good at!

I've noticed many people who are driven feel they must prioritize what they perceive as a weakness, for instance, their speed if they struggle on the track or endurance if they can't maintain their pace for an entire tempo or long run. While I understand the impulse, it's actually counterproductive. If you thrive on certain types of workouts, there's a good chance part of that is because your body responds well to them—and you can take advantage of that.

Of course, you don't want to entirely skip important components of training just because they don't come as naturally to you, but focusing mainly on something you suck at wears you down and saps your confidence. Not only is it not fun, but working against your physiology also means you're not going to see as much progress.

Instead, I recommend a more healthy, holistic, and enjoyable approach to gaining fitness—use your strengths more and dabble in work for your weaknesses.

Here's how it might play out in practice. Say you love mile repeats and tempo runs like I do. Great! Find or create a training plan that includes lots of those! Then every other week or so, balance them out with a workout that focuses on something you're not as good at (in this example, if it's your speed, that'd be a fast track session that gets your legs turning over quickly). That way, you're capitalizing on your strengths without neglecting your weaknesses. You might also think about this when choosing a race—a hilly course allows strength runners to shine, whereas perfect pacers might do better on flat, fast routes.

Through this process, you'll reinforce what's worked for you before so you know which habits to continue. You'll also bring to the surface anything you might need to change or address before you delve into full pursuit of your breakthrough.

PICKING A PLAN

At this point, you have a lot of critical information to guide you as you choose a path from where you are to where you want to be. I have ready-made training plans for distances from 5K to the marathon right here in this book, starting on page 161. But by no means do you have to use them to get value out of these pages. There are plenty of other coaches, websites, books, and magazines that offer training plans, and you might find one that's a better fit for your needs.

Of course, some plans are better than others. It helps to go with a plan from a reputable publication or a credentialed and experienced coach (more on choosing one of those in a minute). Some plans are free and general; others might cost money but in return are individualized to meet your needs.

Regardless of cost, look for a plan that does the following:

- *Starts where you are, not where you hope to be.* Remember that question about your base? Use it here—if you've been running 35 miles per week, jumping immediately into a schedule that demands 60 will likely leave you overtrained or injured.

- *Builds over time at a reasonable rate.* Exactly how rapidly you can safely ramp up depends on many factors. Some coaches recommend the 10 percent rule, whereas others advise adding no more than the number of days you run per week (so if you run six days and rest or cross-train one, you could safely add six miles to your weekly total). If you're frequently injured, you might want to err on the conservative side here.

- *Alternates between days of easy running, faster workouts, and long runs.* Relaxed running is necessary for building a strong base, but you won't reach your full potential without stressing your body through speedwork and longer distances (we'll get into a little more of the science and specifics in chapter 3). Slower running or cross-training allows your body time to recover between long and hard days while still building your aerobic system.

- *Progresses through phases.* Of course, all those elements have to be deployed at the right time to achieve success. Smart coaches design plans based on something called periodization. This is a series of phases in which you'll emphasize a different system or part of your physiology. The exact number and name of these phases vary. My plans have four: stability segment, buildup block, performance phase, and taper time (you'll learn more about them in chapter 11, on page 151).

- *Peaks with a long run of an appropriate distance.* In most cases, your long run should equal or exceed the distance of your goal race. The exception is the marathon (or longer); 26.2 miles is just too taxing to the body to do in practice. (See the next sidebar for more about this.)

- *Uses your strengths.* With so many different plans available, you can likely find one that emphasizes the types of workouts you enjoy while sprinkling in sessions to work on your weaknesses or that have enough flexibility to allow you to tweak on your own. You might also pay a coach to develop a customized or semicustomized plan to tailor an existing schedule to better fit you. This might cost less than full coaching but get you better results than a more generalized plan.

MARATHON MATH

How long is long enough—or too long—for marathon training? The right answer for you might require a little calculating. Most plans max out at 20 or 23 miles, but depending on your pace, you might want to keep them even shorter.

Here's why. Running longer than three hours during a marathon training block breaks your body down too much to repair and train at 100 percent again the next week. So if a 20-plus-mile-long run will take you more than three hours, it's better to make it shorter. In addition, your long run in most instances shouldn't exceed 30 percent of your weekly mileage, so if you want to run 20 miles safely, you should build up to at least 60-mile weeks.

Note, though, this doesn't mean the marathon's off limits for slower or lower-mileage runners. I believe if you can reach a 16-mile-long run during training, you can complete the 26.2-mile distance when you're tapered and rested.

CONSIDER A COACH

So often, runners reach out to me and say they have a goal but don't know whether they're "good enough" or fast enough to hire a coach. You may have even thought this yourself! But if you're looking to improve and you want a partner in the process, you're exactly the type of runner who can, and should, consider coaching. The key is finding the right coach for *you*—and if you're going to make this investment in yourself and your running, you're allowed to be picky.

A quick search online or poll of your running friends will reveal just how many coaches are out there. You can start narrowing your search by checking out their website and social media to see whether what they're saying vibes with you. From there, check out their education, certifications, or experience. There isn't one standard certification process for running coaches, so while you can consider any courses they've taken, it's just as important (if not more so) to look at their experience.

This doesn't just mean their running experience because even though it's ironic coming from me, fast runners don't always make the best coaches. Instead, you'll want to get a sense of types of athletes they've worked with and how successful those partnerships have been. You can read testimonials, look at public team results, or ask for referrals if you like.

From there, ask yourself a few more key questions:

- Do you want a coach who will meet with you in person, or is strictly online OK?
- Do you want other runners to train with—a team-like environment?
- Do you want your coach to check in with you and hold you accountable, or do you prefer a more hands-off approach?
- How frequently do you race, and do you want a coach to talk through strategy and results with you every time?
- Do you prefer a male or female coach, or does it matter?
- Do you feel comfortable taking a plan from a coach and adapting it to your own schedule and needs? Or do you want a coach to adjust your training along the way?
- How much do you want to pay?

Finally, you'll want a coach whose philosophy matches your needs. For instance, some coaches preach high mileage for all their athletes, which won't work if you're a busy, frequently injured runner who knows she needs three days of cross-training per week to stay healthy. If you derive confidence from data, a coach who doesn't bother to look at your splits probably isn't the best fit.

While you can tell a lot from many coaches' websites or social media profiles, it's often best to have an email exchange or phone conversation before you sign up. Share your goals and the basics of your history and lifestyle. You'll want a coach who seems excited about your prospects and has a solid plan for working with your unique circumstances—for understanding your strengths and helping you build on them.

BUILD YOUR TEAM

Even if you don't join a team that meets in person, social runners can build their own training group. Once you start looking for them, prospective training partners are everywhere—on Strava, in group runs from your local running store, on your everyday route. If you thrive on social running like I do, don't be shy about sharing your goal and pulling in others who want to go for it.

Of course, it's also important to consider the other people in your life and how they factor into your ability to achieve your goals. Let's be real—running can be pretty all consuming, and not everyone gets it. If you don't talk to the nonrunners in your life about it, however, they definitely won't understand.

Consider whether you need to have convos with your partner, family, boss, colleagues, or friends about these topics:

- Changes to childcare arrangements
- Financial commitments to coaching, gear, and injury prevention or treatment
- Different eating habits
- Shifts in your regular schedule, for instance, later work hours, longer lunches, or fewer happy hours
- Practical support you might need during training, such as transportation, pacing, or bringing you fuel or water
- Travel time, logistics, and support on race day

Taking the time to explain your goals, why they matter so much, and what you'll need in pursuit of them can go a long way in not only getting you the support you need but also diffusing any tension and frustration along the way. In the best case, you'll turn your ambitions into team efforts—and come up with new ways to return the support you've received.

GEAR UP

It's true that running involves less equipment than most sports, the most critical being a good pair of running shoes. But there are many tools that make life a lot easier when you're going for a big goal. Here are a few purchases to consider:

- A fuel belt, handheld water bottle, or hydration vest for long runs (or instead of carrying water, having another plan, such as stashing water bottles along your route, running a loop, or having someone bring you supplies)
- Recovery and at-home injury management tools (more on these in chapters 3 and 8)
- Home strength-training equipment, such as bands and dumbbells (You'll use these in the exercises in chapter 7, starting on page 98.)
- A treadmill or gym access if you need it because of weather, safety, or childcare constraints

- Reflective or high-visibility items if you're running at dawn or dusk or in the dark
- Clothing appropriate to the weather conditions (If you haven't trained seriously through a northern winter or sweaty summer before, now's the time to ask other runners for advice or hit up your local store for the warmest gloves or sun-shielding hats and visors.)
- A watch with the functions you want (Because GPS or smart watches are often expensive, if you're making this investment, do your research to ensure the one you purchase offers the features you plan to use. For instance, if you want to program in your workouts, an Apple Watch or Fitbit won't cut it—you'll need a Garmin, COROS, Polar, or something similar. If you train by heart rate, you'll need to add a chest strap—not just the wrist data from the watch, which is less accurate.)
- About those running shoes: By now, you probably have an idea of what type of shoe works best for you; if you don't, your local running shop is a great place to get personalized advice and find a pair that feels comfortable. While it's easy to get overwhelmed by shoe technology and lingo, many biomechanics experts say shoe comfort is the most important variable in running your best and avoiding injury (Nigg et al. 2015).

Keep in mind that you should replace your shoes approximately every 300 to 350 miles to reduce your injury risk and that just one pair won't take you through a whole marathon-training cycle. Many runners find it helpful to have two pairs of shoes they're alternating—depending on your physiology and distance, this might be a cushier pair for longer runs and a lighter-weight or carbon fiber–plate shoe for racing and workouts. One last pro tip: If you find a brand and model you like, don't be afraid to stock up on them so you don't fall in love only to find them discontinued the next time you're due for a new pair!

TAKE NOTES

As the questions in this chapter make clear, the more information you have about the training you've done in the past, the more guidance you have for your future. That's why I strongly recommend keeping a detailed training log.

I personally keep both digital and paper records. My watch data uploads to Strava and Final Surge, but I also write down everything in my *Believe Training Journal* (Fleshman and McGettigan-Dumas 2014). And when I say everything, I mean far more than just my mileage and splits. I include notes about how my body felt that day, my mood, the small steps I took toward my goals. (This particular journal, written by former pro runners Lauren Fleshman and Roisin McGettigan-Dumas, is full of helpful prompts and tips. It makes the whole process simpler—and a lot more fun.)

That way, I have a snapshot of not only my physical preparation but also my mindset. I can review the way I trained for a particular course—strengthening my quads in the gym and on declines for the hills of Boston—so I have a blueprint for how to do it again without excess soreness. But I can also recapture what I was thinking and feeling heading into a big race. Based on the outcome, I'll know where to place my mental focus next time. Hindsight also helps me spot patterns I want to change—say, the days I ran through foot pain that later turned into weeks off.

Flipping back through the pages of your log immediately before a race can give you a huge confidence boost. Deena Kastor famously highlights her breakthrough training runs in pink and yellow. That way, when doubts creep into her mind, she can quickly and visually remind herself of all the work she's put in and what she's already accomplished (Kuzma 2015).

Life Lessons: Tina Muir

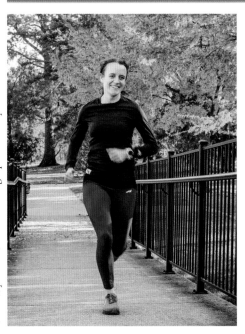

Courtesy of Tina Muir. Photographer: Sandy Gutierrez.

As a young girl in England, Tina Muir hated running enough to hide in the bathroom during cross country tryouts. But something convinced her to join the school's team and eventually, a local club, and by the time she was a teenager, she was placing in the top 20 nationally and was hungry for more.

She came to the United States for college, and her performance shifted into high gear when she landed at Ferris State University in Michigan. "I was thrown into a situation where everyone took their training so seriously," she says. From daily practice to races that required 14-hour road trips, the intensity of the environment awoke her inner competitor. "I felt an immense pressure to prove myself and was determined to be at the front of the team."

And she succeeded, finishing 12th at her first national cross country championship a year later, but before too long, success took a toll. She ran alone, deeming the team too slow, and began pushing herself too hard while fueling too little. She alternated between cycles of injury and recovery, never truly finding stability.

"I got better, but marginally, and more and more felt like I was just a runner, with nothing else to add to the world," she says. Though she loved the sport, she hated the pressure that came with it—stress that, though she couldn't see it at the time, came largely from within.

Working with a sport psychologist, Evie Serventi, helped Tina finally peel back the pressure and remind her of the joy she'd originally found on the cross country course. She signed up for the London Marathon in 2015, her third go at the distance, and though she once again missed her goal of 2:40 by about a minute, she placed seventh and smiled the whole way.

Soon after, her long-held dreams fell into place. At age 28, she competed for Great Britain and Northern Ireland in the World Half Marathon Championships and, five weeks later, ran a personal-best 2:37 at the 2016 London Marathon. She then bettered that mark at the California International Marathon in December, where she ran a 2:36:39.

But in the end, she realized the lifestyle wasn't sustainable for her. "I love to run, but I also love to do a lot of other things," she says. "As hard as I tried, I could not juggle the intensity of training at the top level with all the other life experiences and goals I had in other areas. I experienced burnout over and over again, and it did not feel good. My health took a toll and so did my heart."

She quit the sport in 2017 and started a family. Today, most people know Tina as host of the *Running for Real* and *Running Realized* podcasts; the mother of Bailey and Chloe; and the creator of a thriving community dedicated to fostering a healthy mindset about running and training. Too often, she believes, runners at all levels are shown only one path, the one that leads to "paces and splits, races and extrinsic rewards."

She hopes, instead, to reconnect them to emotions such as joy, appreciation, and self-compassion. Dreaming big can empower us, she believes, but only if we show ourselves kindness along the way.

"It is amazing that you are going for a big goal. I am excited for you and will be a part of your cheering squad, but I also want you to see that this big goal accomplishment is not going to change who you are for better or for worse," she says. "Things will go wrong, and life will throw curveballs. But remember, it is all part of the journey, part of that growth. The finish line is the celebration, but the best part is the training and what you learn about yourself along the way."

FROM BARRIER TO BREAKTHROUGH

If you've done every exercise in this chapter, you might already have a list of process goals. Nearly every runner embarking on a big goal can make the Know Yourself assessment on page 15 a first priority. But here are a few other ideas for overcoming obstacles early in your planning and training process.

Barrier

I'm lost when it comes to finding the best training plan for me.

Breakthrough Goals

Choose one or more.

I will do the following:

- Take a look at the plans that begin in chapter 11, page 154, to see whether they might be right for me
- Compare a few plans from magazines, books, or websites to see whether they meet my needs
- Think about hiring a coach to design a plan for me

Barrier

I'm curious about hiring a coach but not sure where to start.

Breakthrough Goals

Choose one or more.

I will do the following:

- Make a list of what I want from a coach
- Do a search and ask other runners I know to find prospective coaches
- Schedule calls with one or more coaches to see whether their philosophy aligns with my needs

---

Barrier

I'm not sure whether I can reach this big goal on my own.

Breakthrough Goals

Choose one or more.

I will do the following:

- Look into finding a coach who has a training group
- Recruit some training partners
- Talk to my friends, family, colleagues, and anyone else in my life about the support I need

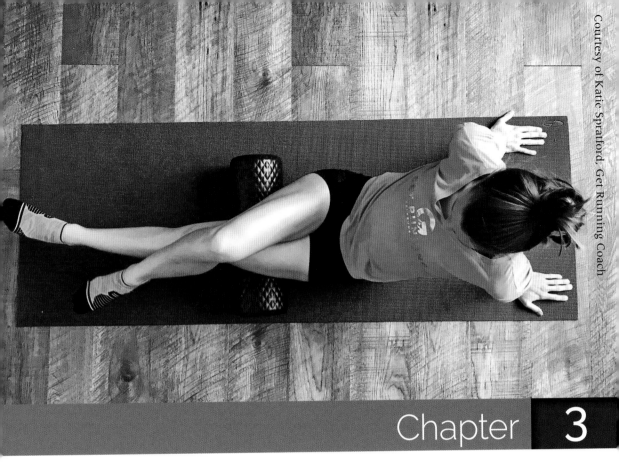

Courtesy of Katie Spratford, Get Running Coach

Chapter **3**

Recover Right

" The grind can become your weakness if you plow through so many little problems that you suddenly have . . . really stubborn, work-hardened problems. We can be so good at not letting anything get in our way, unless it's our own dang self trying to train through too much. Sometimes, it feels like a step back to figure it out or rest, but cross-training, body work, and recovery are still inching you along to the performance goal. "

Molly Huddle, two-time Olympian and 10,000-meter American record holder

You might think it's your training alone that leads to progress. While it's true your workouts provide the stimulus to adapt, it's the time between sessions when the true magic happens. That's when your body repairs and rebuilds you into a stronger, fitter, more efficient runner.

Brad Stulberg and Steve Magness provide a simple description of all this in their book *Peak Performance* and on their website The Growth Equation: stress + rest = growth (Stulberg and Magness 2017). (Magness also happens to be one of my former coaches!) Striking the right balance between these variables is essential in reaching your goals and preventing burnout and injury. In this chapter, we'll focus on enhancing your recovery so you can truly reap the benefits of all your hard work.

A RECOVERY REVELATION

As a pro runner, I have plenty of experience with physical therapists, chiropractors, and orthopedic specialists, and like most moms, see my obstetrician and pediatrician more often than some of my family members. But my one and only visit to an urgent care center came because I had severely neglected recovery.

To back up a bit, the "rest" half of the growth equation has never come easy for me. In high school, my nickname was Energizer Bunny. I'd go nonstop from morning until night, from class to practice to races, and then do it all over again.

I carried a similar "work hard, then work harder" mindset into college and beyond. That worked well enough for me when my primary focus was only on training and racing, but as my other responsibilities increased, what little recovery I was doing became even more of an afterthought. Getting pregnant with Athens required me to take time off from running, but I channeled those hours into building my coaching business. I'm not proud of this, but I actually started working from the hospital the day after I delivered, laptop on one side and a new, nursing baby on the other.

Of course, having a child only added more responsibilities to my to-do list, from changing diapers to getting my body back in shape. Other people started noticing how much pressure I was putting on myself. Some suggested techniques such as meditation, which I promptly blew off. Didn't they realize how *busy* I was?

Finally, just after Athens' first birthday, I hit a breaking point. First, I fractured my hip on a run. My left hip had been hurting for a while thanks to postpartum hormonal shifts, but I'd sought treatment and was on the mend. Then at mile 13 of a 14-mile effort, I felt a sharp, stabbing pain on my right side. This came completely out of nowhere—I'd had zero symptoms at all in this area. As I hobbled around afterward (eventually, an MRI confirmed a fracture), my mind filled with doubts and fears about the future. *Had I completely lost touch with my body? Was my career over?*

The icing on the cake came when Athens was teething and waking up for the day at 3:00 a.m. for weeks in a row. Through it all, I kept pushing—until I couldn't. My energy levels tanked. I could barely get out of bed in the morning, let alone out the door to exercise.

My typically sunny personality dulled into a mild despair. Things that once brought me joy left me feeling numb instead. One day, I took Athens to the water park with friends. Normally, I'd be laughing with my fellow moms as we splashed, jumped, and played in the spray, a welcome relief from the hot Colorado sun. But this time, all I wanted to do was go home and be alone. I still have a photo from that day, and while Athens looks happy and adorable, it reflects nothing of how I felt inside.

After a few weeks of this, I asked a neighbor for help watching Athens, and the three of us headed to urgent care. I was certain I'd be diagnosed with mono or maybe even pneumonia. Four hours and multiple tests later, doctors told me it wasn't a virus or bacteria that had laid me so low—it was sheer exhaustion.

My prescription? A daily 30-minute dose of restoration. I began blocking a half hour into my schedule during which I wasn't allowed to coach, mom, or train. I might call a friend; take a nap; watch an episode or two of *Modern Love*; bake some muffins; or read some sports romance from one of my favorite authors, Ali Dean—anything that rebooted my system.

After two weeks, I felt like myself again. Only then could I recommit to the rehab and training that would get me past my hip injury and back into elite shape.

Do I think my hard-charging personality has helped me succeed as a runner? Absolutely. But this extreme example made it crystal clear: I must work equally hard on prioritizing rest. And although this is not the most compelling example, when I look back through my years of training, most of my regrets have to do with pushing through when I probably should have backed off or rested more.

When you're asking your body to do things it's never done before, it's more essential than ever to allow it time and space to meet the challenge. Skip the recovery, and at best, you won't benefit as much from your training. At worst, you'll stress your body beyond the point when repair and restoration are possible and wind up injured, over-trained, or so wiped out you'll swear you have a serious infection.

BUILDING YOUR ENGINE

My hope is to convince you of the critical importance of rest and recovery, minus any unnecessary medical visits! Understanding a bit about how your body responds to hard efforts can make it easier to honor your need to recuperate.

For distances of 5K and longer—in fact, for any event that lasts longer than three minutes—the most important element of training is developing the aerobic system. If you've ever started a training block feeling winded after three or four miles, then built up to comfortably run 10- or 20-mile distances, you understand what gaining aerobic fitness feels like.

Training the aerobic system is all about getting vital oxygen to your hard-working muscles as quickly as possible. On the run itself, you're putting stress on your system, increasing the demands on your heart and lungs as well as your legs. During the recovery process, your body adapts to handle that extra strain so you can push even harder the next time. So in the hours and days between runs, you may think you're resting—but that's truly when the gains occur.

During recovery, the following processes occur:

- Your heart—and especially your left ventricle—grows larger and stronger, to pump more oxygen-rich blood out with each beat.

- Production of red blood cells and hemoglobin, a protein within the cells on which oxygen molecules hitch a ride, ramps up.

- You'll sprout more capillaries around your muscle cells, so more fresh blood flows in—and waste products, such as carbon dioxide, easily flush out.

- Inside those muscle cells, your body builds more—and larger—mitochondria. These mini factories use oxygen to turn glycogen and fatty acids into ATP (adenosine triphosphate), a fuel that powers every contraction.

- As your muscles run out of the glycogen stores inside them, they'll replenish to a higher level. At the same time, your body becomes more efficient at burning fat too—especially important in longer distances, such as the marathon (Murray et al. 2016).

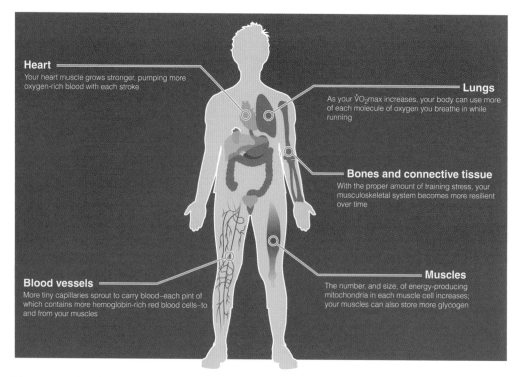

Heart
Your heart muscle grows stronger, pumping more oxygen-rich blood with each stroke

Lungs
As your V̇O₂max increases, your body can use more of each molecule of oxygen you breathe in while running

Bones and connective tissue
With the proper amount of training stress, your musculoskeletal system becomes more resilient over time

Blood vessels
More tiny capillaries sprout to carry blood—each pint of which contains more hemoglobin-rich red blood cells—to and from your muscles

Muscles
The number, and size, of energy-producing mitochondria in each muscle cell increases; your muscles can also store more glycogen

How your body adapts to aerobic training

On top of all that, you're applying stress to your musculoskeletal system—inflicting just enough minor damage to your muscles, bones, and connective tissue so they repair and become more resilient structures.

Your running provides a stimulus that jump-starts all these processes. However, it's in the hours and days off the track or path—and, especially, when you're asleep—that most of them occur.

SIX TYPES OF RECOVERY

I'm using the word *recovery* to mean everything that happens when your body isn't under serious stress, whether it's from a hard workout, a work presentation, or a confrontation with your significant other. Because it's such a broad term, I find it helpful to consider the various forms it can take.

- *Recovery runs.* Easy miles offer an opportunity to continue building aerobic fitness without overtaxing your body.
- *Active recovery.* Strategic time on the bike or elliptical, in the pool, or even briskly walking—anything that's low intensity and less than 45 minutes—gets your blood flowing to bathe your insides with recovery hormones, even as these activities slightly boost your aerobic system.
- *Passive recovery.* Activities that offer you a sense of relaxation and restoration, from deep breathing to watching reality TV to connecting with friends and family, fall into this category.

- *Assisted recovery.* Many tools and techniques—some convenient and inexpensive enough for the average athlete to use at home and others higher tech and costly—promise to accelerate the process by which training adaptations occur so you're ready to run hard again. These include compression boots, cupping sets, and massage guns.
- *Sleep.* Study after study makes it clear: sleep is essential to nearly all of the adaptations discussed so far (Vitale et al. 2019; Watson et al. 2017). It's the closest thing we have to a miracle recovery method.
- *Scheduled downtime.* I recommend runners take some time away between training cycles—at least one to two full weeks off at least twice per year. Legendary athletes say this has been integral to their careers, offering them a chance to reset their mind and body before they lock into their next big goal.

You might notice you're better at some of these than others, but they're all things you can work to improve if you find yourself needing more recovery.

RECOVERY ON THE RUN

I'll admit that, early in my running career, recovery runs weren't a part of my repertoire. In true Energizer Bunny style, I rarely slowed below a seven-minute pace.

But then I moved to Colorado in 2015 and went for a run with Kara Goucher, an accomplished athlete I'd long looked up to. We ran 11 miles at 8:30 pace—definitely speedy, but relatively speaking, it was more than two and a half minutes slower than the pace I'd run the entire 26.2-mile Boston Marathon the next year. My first thought was, *What are we doing?* That was closely followed by this realization: *I feel amazing!*

I asked whether she often ran this slowly. She pointed out that she'd had a hard workout the day before and a long, hard run the next day in the middle of a 100-plus-mile week. Without these easy efforts, her system wouldn't be able to take the strain.

The experience shifted my entire mindset. I'd long known that workouts and long runs each had a specific purpose, but now I began to internalize the fact that easy days did, too, and were just as crucial to my development as an athlete.

I started purposely scheduling recovery runs with friends in the neighborhood who weren't pro runners so I wouldn't be tempted to push the pace. I'd sometimes wear a heart rate monitor, using it to hold myself back from going too fast. Slowing down allowed me to put more of my effort into my workouts and was key to achieving all I did at Boston, New York, and beyond.

You'll see in chapters 12 through 15 that my training plans have at least two recovery runs per week. Some refer to them as "junk miles," but I assure you, they have tremendous value. Plus, I never stack two hard workouts or long runs back-to-back.

Some runners may find they need even more recovery to train their hardest; for instance, I have athletes who train on nine- instead of seven-day schedules. They might wind up doing a long run on Thursday of one week and Saturday of the next, but the upside is that they always have two easy days between hard workouts.

SOME DAYS OFF

"No days off" might work well as a meme or a marketing slogan, but for most runners, it's not practical. Those who aren't elites (and even some who are) typically don't have either the optimal biomechanics or ample hours for recovery. At any one time, I might have about 5 out of 80 or more athletes I coach—and remember, this includes

SLOW YOUR ROLL

Many runners have a harder time slowing down than they do hitting fast paces. One way to stay honest is to calculate your target paces and aim for those. You can use the charts on page 157 for help.

If you're still having a hard time taking it easy enough, you can do the following:

- *Buddy up.* Try my technique of running with (preferably, slower) friends and catching up on the run. If you can't talk, you're running way too fast!
- *"Paws" often.* Take your dog and stop whenever nature calls or a good smell requires a sniff.
- *Hit the trail.* Try a more scenic route than usual and focus on relaxing enough to take in the view.
- *Breathe easy.* I'll explain more about how to focus on your breath in chapter 10, on page 139. But in brief, extend your inhales and exhales, counting to four for each. Slow your strides to match this rhythm.
- *Track your ticker.* Wear a heart rate monitor (a chest strap is better—it measures the actual electrical activity of your heart, whereas watches use a less precise measure of reflected light). You can look up formulas to calculate your maximum heart rate and all the zones underneath, but I prefer to start by measuring heart rate at prescribed paces for a few weeks, then averaging out the number. My aerobic pace, for instance, is 130 to 140. Yours may be higher or lower, but once you've calibrated it, you can aim to stay within it.

competitive runners who are qualifying for the Olympic Marathon Trials—who run seven days a week.

Nine out of 10 times, my athletes take one complete day off—no exercise at all. If they must move, I'll recommend a yoga class, a swim, or an easy bike ride, preferably something that doesn't involve an elevated heart rate or high impact. This regular day of off-loading further enhances recovery and also allows time for minor tweaks to heal before they become injuries.

THE WHOLE STRESS PIE

Your body has a finite amount of energy that it uses to accomplish everything in your life. It's hard to run your best when things are hectic at work, with your family, or in other areas. While this makes sense on its face, it's often hard for athletes to understand—or admit—the way external stressors can affect them.

Sometimes, it can help to simply write out all your sources of stress. I recently did this with a coaching client who was disappointed with his paces. He wrote down a lengthy list of things that were wearing him out—a new baby, a pandemic, a busy period at work, and summer's heat and humidity. When he compared this list to where he was a year ago, only the heat and humidity had remained constant. It was then easy for him to see why running felt harder at the moment.

Another way to make this real is to draw out your "stress pie." Think of the amount of energy you have as a full circle, like a pie chart. Divide it into slices that represent everything you have going on in your life. You can swiftly see that a busy time that requires one slice to grow (such as a huge project at work that has you up late at night) or even adds a new slice (such as a move or a new baby) can decrease the amount of energy your body has to train well and adapt to that training.

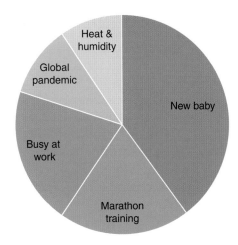

Possible stressors in a runner's life

There's some more advice about minimizing the effect of stressors in chapter 9, on page 128. Adding in extra recovery, even if it changes the timeline you had in mind for making your breakthrough, is one of the best things you can do for your running, not to mention your health and well-being.

THE SCIENCE OF SLUMBER

When we're crunched for time, sleep is often the first thing we sacrifice. However, it's not a risk worth taking. Take it from a sleep expert—Shelby Harris, PsyD, a licensed clinical psychologist board certified in behavioral sleep medicine by the American Academy of Sleep Medicine and the author of *The Women's Guide to Overcoming Insomnia: Get a Good Night's Sleep without Relying on Medication*. While you're "resting," these processes occur:

- Your pituitary gland secretes human growth hormone, a potent biochemical that strengthens bones, repairs muscles, and converts fat into fuel.
- Your glycogen stores replenish.
- Your body repairs micro-damage to your tissues, decreasing your injury risk and speeding healing if you do get hurt.
- Signals between your brain and body are encoded into muscle memory.
- Your immune system strengthens, reducing your risk of illness.

When you're well rested, your emotional regulation also improves, meaning you think better, remember more, and tolerate higher levels of stress. All of this is extremely helpful for balancing running and life.

When Harris—a marathoner herself—is aiming for a big goal, such as a Boston-qualifying time, she makes sleep an even higher priority and diligently plans how she'll get enough of it. "Is every night perfect? No. But I know that I get way more benefit from my training program if sleep is a key component, along with a healthy diet," she says.

The American Academy of Sleep Medicine and the Sleep Research Society recommend the average adult sleep at least seven hours per night. When you're training hard, you might need even more. Stress, a packed schedule, and caffeine can interfere with a runners' rest; hormones can also disrupt sleep during menopause, perimenopause (which starts in your 40s), and even just before your period. And of course, once kids come into the picture, their own fragmented sleep schedules affect you too.

Harris' advice to busy runners includes the following:

- Wind down for at least 30 to 60 minutes before bedtime with a book, music, art, or meditation. "Sleep isn't an on-off switch," she says. Time away from the blue light of screens, plus a relaxing routine, allows your brain to settle into it. And if you are on your computer or tablet later in the day, consider blue light glasses, which can minimize the effects of these rays on your body's production of the sleep hormone melatonin (Shecter et al. 2018).

- Power naps—about 20 minutes long—can help in a pinch, but don't take them after 2:00 p.m. Also, lay off caffeine after that time. Its effects can linger for hours and interrupt deep sleep.

- Generally, a steady schedule—keeping the same bedtime and waking time every day—is best. But if your main trouble is fitting adequate sleep into your schedule, you can tinker with banking an extra hour or two of rest by sleeping in on the weekends or on days off from running. (Just be prepared to abandon this tactic if you start having trouble falling or staying asleep, she warns.)

- Get help when you need it. If you struggle with sleep for weeks or months on end, despite your efforts to address it, or if it comes paired with other symptoms, such as hot flashes or a racing mind, talk to your doctor or find a sleep medicine specialist. "There are really good treatments out there, many of which don't require medication," she says.

LEVEL UP YOUR RECOVERY

There's no substitute for adequate sleep, but certain tools and techniques may fast-forward the recovery process. These include the following:

- *Compression boots.* Popular brands include Normatec and Rapid Reboot. By inflating and deflating air pockets along your legs, you'll boost blood flow and carry away the metabolic waste products your body produces during hard efforts. You can find them at some gyms, athlete lounges, and physical therapist's offices, or you can pick up your own pair for around $1,000.

- *Compression garments.* Snug-fitting compression socks, tights, or leg sleeves lack mechanical action but still help when you wear them during or after a hard workout. Plus, they come at a much more reasonable price. Wear them traveling to and from a race to reduce the risk of blood clots, which can occur when you're cramped in a car or plane seat (Clarke et al. 2016).

- *Heat therapy.* Research suggests that either heat or cold can reduce muscle soreness after hard efforts, so experiment and see what feels better for you (Petrofsky et al. 2015).

RECOVERY DIET

We'll talk a lot more about fueling your performance in chapter 4, but eating for recovery warrants a quick mention here. Hydration is critical, both throughout the day and during and after your runs. Soon after a race or a hard workout—within about 30 minutes—you'll want a snack with both carbohydrate and protein. Carbohydrate begins replenishing depleted glycogen stores, whereas protein is essential for repairing muscle damage. In fact, while runners often associate protein primarily with strength training, endurance athletes also need plenty throughout the day.

I love doing some light stretching in the hot tub or yoga in the sauna after a race. You'll just want to limit how long you spend there—maybe 10 minutes, max—and drink plenty of water. If you don't have access to one of those hot spots, dump a few cups of Epsom salts—readily available at any drugstore—into a warm bathtub.

- *Ice baths.* All you need here is cold water, some ice cubes, and a tub. As with heat, about 10 minutes works well to reduce inflammation and enhance recovery. There's some evidence that hopping back and forth between heat and cold works even better at shuttling blood and waste products through your system (Shadgan et al. 2018).

- *Hot or cold compresses.* When you don't have the time—or space—for a full dunk, spot treat particularly sore or tight areas. One of my favorite recent discoveries is IceeNOW Instant Wraps, which combine cold therapy with compression, no freezer required.

- *Massage or self-massage.* Foam rollers; percussive massagers, such as the RePro by Ultra Recovery; or the trained hands of a massage therapist can aid recovery and ward off injury (more about this in chapter 8, on page 121).

I'd recommend these methods before or after hard workouts or races, especially in your peak phase of training or if you're frequently traveling or racing.

POSTRACE RESTORATION

On race day—especially if it's your goal race—you're leaving it all on the line. Asking a lot of your body means you'll need to flip the switch and prioritize recovery above all else on the other side.

First things first—after a race of any distance, drink plenty of fluids to rehydrate and include electrolytes, which are valuable minerals, such as sodium and potassium, that you lose through sweat. (When a postrace volunteer hands you a bottle of Gatorade, take it or pack your own sports drink of choice.) You'll also want protein to repair muscle damage. And then, of course, there's the celebratory treats that help us revel in our accomplishments—the brew from the beer tent, burger and fries, or ice cream sundae.

Traveling? If you're taking a particularly long flight, wear compression boots or garments, stay hydrated, and consider taking a baby aspirin 30 minutes before takeoff to prevent blood clots. Get up frequently and walk the aisle to the bathroom. If you're driving, stop at least every hour or so to stretch your legs.

For races of half-marathon distance or shorter, stick to easy runs for a few days afterward, then work back into training. For a marathon or longer, it's a good idea to build in complete rest days. After my hardest efforts, I've stopped running for a full two weeks in favor of active recovery, especially in the pool. Assisted recovery tools and techniques—from ice baths to steam rooms to massages (I always schedule mine two to four days after, when my body's already beginning the repair process)—can also help at this time.

Above all, listen to your body and stay cautious—immediately after a race, it's all too easy to dig yourself into a deeper hole. After the Houston Marathon in 2020, I had hoped to bounce back quickly and run the Olympic Marathon Trials six weeks later. I quickly realized the toll the 26.2-mile distance took on my body. Begrudgingly, I shut down the thought of training and took a two-week reset.

I headed into the Trials knowing I wouldn't be ready to finish the race. While I was disappointed, I knew it wasn't worth risking a longer-term injury or setback. By now, I'm patient enough to know that, when my body's ready, my next breakthrough will come.

RATE YOUR RECOVERY

While there are some rules of thumb—seven hours of sleep per night, one day off a week, at least one recovery run in between hard efforts—each runner's exact recipe for success varies. Plus, your needs change as your training load increases, with age, and based on other stressors in your life. These monitoring methods can help you keep tabs and continue striking the right balance.

Resting Heart Rate

This simple self-check requires only a watch or the clock on your phone. First thing in the morning, count your pulse for 30 seconds. (Note: If you often wake up with a full bladder, experiment with getting up and emptying it first, getting back into bed, and taking a few deep breaths. As I've learned firsthand, having to pee is a stress that can increase your heart rate.) Double this number, then write it down—that's your resting heart rate, or RHR.

While the American Heart Association notes that a healthy range is 60 to 100, athletes' RHR can be as low as the upper 30s. Once you start monitoring, you'll get a feel for your baseline. From there, you can take action when you notice fluctuations. If your heart rate is 10 beats per minute or higher above your norm, I recommend doing an easy run instead of a workout that day. Up 20 beats per minute? Consider taking a complete rest day.

This number can tell you all kinds of other interesting things too! Your RHR tends to rise at altitude, when you're about to get sick, around the time of your period or ovulation, and during pregnancy. You'll probably notice it's higher when you come back to training after a break and slightly decreases as your fitness improves with training.

Mood and Motivation

This is slightly less scientific and more subjective but still telling. If you're suddenly feeling lackluster about your goals, dreading your training, or not having fun most days, you might be underrecovered.

This is where a training log with room for notes, such as the *Believe* journal, or a digital log, such as Final Surge, which allows you to color-code each day of training (green is good, yellow average, red poor) comes in. We all have an off day here and there. But if you're consistently describing your workouts as disappointing, finding the word *ugh* written over and over, or seeing a string of red days with little green, try adding extra recovery.

Heart Rate Variability

This one's for the data geeks and requires some technology. Your heart rate variability, or HRV, measures how much the time between your heartbeats varies, in milliseconds. Unlike RHR, which we want to stay steady, HRV fluctuates in rhythm with our efforts. In fact, these shifts tell us we're training appropriately and not overburdening our nervous system.

Some GPS watches track your HRV, as do tools such as the WHOOP strap or ithlete, a finger sensor that attaches to your phone. A high number is a green light, a sign that your body's recovered and ready for a hard effort. The day after a workout, you'll notice lower readings.

Using HRV provides a more complete and nuanced picture of the total amount of stress you're under and whether your body's up to the task of recovering from it. I find it works particularly well if you work night shifts or have a stressful schedule, trouble listening to your body's cues of fatigue, or have had problems with burnout or over-training before.

The key to any of these measures, however, is acting on the information you're given. Sensors such as WHOOP and ithlete give you detailed recommendations on when to completely rest or switch to an easy run and when it's OK to proceed with a planned workout. This requires flexibility and a basic knowledge of how to manipulate the days of your training plan or a coach who can adjust your schedule for you.

RECOVERY TO THE RESCUE

Building in recovery runs on a regular basis can help keep you on the right side of the stress–rest equation. Still, ambitious athletes may overshoot and find themselves struggling to adequately recover. And as was the case for me before my slightly embarrassing urgent care visit, there are times when other sources of stress deplete the body's resources.

If you find yourself in this position, don't panic—that's counterproductive. But do pay attention to early warning signs, such as flagging motivation or a rise in RHR. As soon as you spot a pattern, I recommend taking one full week to run only easy recovery miles. You won't lose any fitness whatsoever, and your body will have the chance to completely reset and start the next week refreshed.

I have some athletes who have found this technique so powerful that we've built it into their training schedules. They might do 40 to 50 miles weekly with a workout and a long run for three weeks—then on the fourth, just 25 miles, split into five easy five-mile runs. If you don't have a coach individually directing you, you can easily start any training plan early and add in down weeks throughout it.

Still a doubter? Just ask my dad, who attributes one of his greatest athletic achievements to this strategy ("Recovery Pace for Runners ([With Guest Speaker Steve Spence]). In 1990, he was supposed to run the Chicago Marathon in October. But after a strong performance at the Philadelphia Marathon in mid-September, "the wheels came off," as he describes it. Allergies began interfering with his breathing and raising his heart rate, hampering his recovery.

He backed out of Chicago and spent three weeks running only easy miles. He wore a heart rate monitor and kept his efforts to a maximum of 140 to 150 beats per minute. That rest—plus a cold snap that put a freeze on the allergens in the air—turned everything around. His pace at that heart rate dropped about a minute, from seven- to six-minute miles, and he knew he might be ready to race (Burfoot 2020).

On November 11, he ran the Columbus Marathon, which doubled as the U.S. Championships. His goal was to finish without walking, but he wound up winning with a personal-best 2:12:16. To this day, he calls it his best race ever—and it earned him a trip to the World Championships in Tokyo the next year, where he claimed a bronze medal in brutally hot conditions (Spence 2011).

Slow, Steady Victories: Molly Huddle

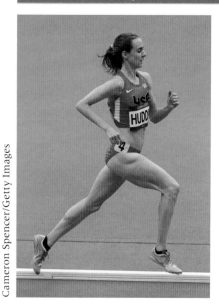

Cameron Spencer/Getty Images

By the time she graduated from Notre Dame, Molly Huddle was used to working hard—and running fast. She was a 10-time All-American and the runner-up in the 5,000 meters at the 2006 NCAA Outdoor Track and Field Championships.

The one thing she wasn't good at was downtime. "I thought I was superwoman and just wasn't aware of how much recovery I needed," she says. She kept herself in what she calls a "gray zone" of mediocre workouts and mediocre recovery. "I would run a little too hard, and I always packed my day to the point of not sleeping enough or being a little too stressed."

Within weeks of graduating, Molly kicked off her pro career by joining a group of women from her new Providence, Rhode Island–based team as they raced in Europe. In races and workouts, "they were all kicking my butt," Molly recalls. But for as hard as they worked, she also noted how slow they ran their easy runs and how they seemed almost "lazy" outside of their training.

Molly decided to learn from them and followed their example. That month, she set personal bests in three events and felt better than she ever had. "I knew it wasn't from new training, as I was only a month removed from my college days," she says. "With adequate recovery, I was running times that probably could have won NCAAs a few weeks earlier."

Though she wishes she'd absorbed this lesson earlier, she's carried it with her throughout her professional career. In addition to hard track workouts and marathon-training long runs, she incorporates yoga, swimming, massage, and chiropractic visits. At the end of each season, once or twice per year, she takes two weeks off entirely, then two to three more weeks of rebuilding mileage before adding in hard workouts.

The results speak for themselves. She's claimed national championships at distances from 5K to 20K, made two Olympic teams, and broken American records on the track and the roads. Now, in mid-2021, she has a personal-best marathon time of 2:26:44 and still holds the American record at 10,000 meters and the half marathon.

As her career has evolved, she's continued to fine-tune her stress–rest equation. "Some seasons I feel like I can inch the workload up, and I absorb more and more, whereas other seasons I feel like I'm not handling the load as well," she says. In addition to the race she's preparing for, the amount of recovery she needs depends on such factors as whether she's training at altitude and the amount of stress in the rest of her life. "One bad workout every few weeks is normal, but a rough month or so is usually a sign of needing more recovery. I have to remind myself that I get fit quick enough, so if it's not happening, it's usually lack of recovery, not lack of work, that is the problem."

Age plays a role too. As she progresses through her third decade, Molly notices herself continuing to reevaluate. She can still go for big goals—but must incorporate even more recovery, cross-training, or injury-prevention work. She looks to athletes who've performed well in their late 30s—Jo Pavey, Edna Kiplagat, Meb Keflezighi, and Shalane Flanagan—for advice and inspiration.

Her advice to other runners, at every age, is to place a premium on recovery. If you have a bad race or workout, consider whether you truly need to press harder—or if in fact, you need to add rest instead. "Often recovery is overlooked as a solution, especially recovery between workouts. It's very common to run recovery mileage too hard," she says. "Lack of recovery is insidious because you can get so used to being tired that you don't know what workouts and races actually should feel like until something makes you slow down!" Her hope is that you can take her cue and chill out to go faster before an injury or another setback forces the issue.

FROM BARRIER TO BREAKTHROUGH

Being just as deliberate and intentional about recovery as you are about your training can allow you to truly take your fitness to the next level. Here are some ideas to help you make it a habit.

Barrier

Every time I near the peak of my training plan, I start to crumble.

Breakthrough Goals

Choose one or more.

I will do the following:

- Slow down on my recovery runs—perhaps by running with a friend, a dog, or a heart rate monitor
- Add in one extra day of recovery per week
- Build in an extra week with lower mileage and only recovery running between peak-mileage weeks
- Block 30 minutes to one hour into my schedule every day for passive recovery—something just for me

_____

Barrier

I know I need more sleep but just can't find the time.

Breakthrough Goals

Choose one or more.

I will do the following:

- Inventory everything I do in the hour before bedtime and see what can be rescheduled so I hit the hay earlier (If an hour is overwhelming, start with 10 minutes at a time.)
- Try to get an extra hour or two on the weekends or days off from running if it doesn't interfere with my ability to drift off
- Try to get my kid(s) on a steady sleep schedule and plan my own around it (It won't be perfect every day, and I might end up getting up in the night. But consistent bedtimes are good for both little ones and grown-up runners!)

_____

Barrier

I'm falling short of my goals despite trying my best, but I'm not sure whether recovery is my problem.

Breakthrough Goals

Choose one or more.

I will do the following:

- Start taking my resting heart rate every morning, noting trends over time, and adding extra recovery if it rises
- Write notes about my mood and motivation levels in my training log and see whether they're on the decline
- Invest in a WHOOP strap or ithlete sensor and begin adjusting my training schedule based on heart rate variability

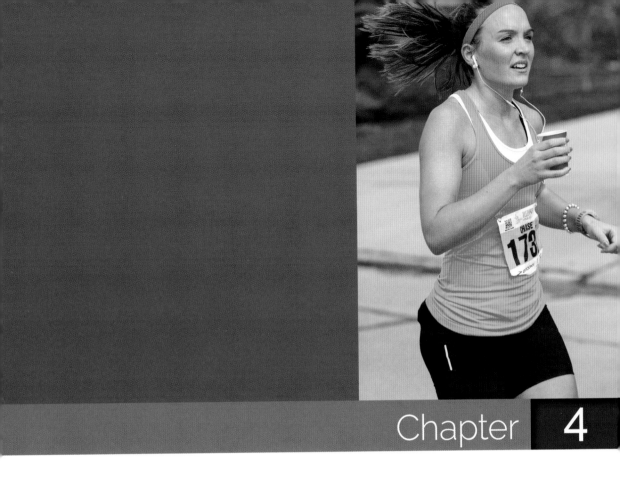

Chapter 4

Feed Your Fire

❝ Eating less isn't how you become a better runner. Consistently nourishing your body is how you become a strong one. ❞

Starla Garcia, dietitian, Olympic Trials marathoner, and body and cultural diversity advocate

Nutrition plays a huge role in your success as an athlete. If you want to run your best, you can't restrict your energy; rather, you need to supply your body with ample ingredients to recover and reap the results of your training.

Each runner has a different recipe for a sustainable, healthy eating plan. However, a few basic principles can help you determine how much, what, and when to eat. That includes how to fuel during training runs and races so you stay energized from the starting line through your finishing kick.

SUCCESS FOR THE LONG RUN

Running requires a lot of your body, and food is the fuel that powers you through every workout, provides the raw materials to rebuild muscles and connective tissue, and drives you toward your goals. Nutrition is also an emotionally fraught issue that can feel confusing, overwhelming, and demoralizing. As runners and women, we get mixed messages from the sport and from society at large about how to eat and drink and how our bodies "should" look to be healthy and to perform our best. And when we set big goals, the desire to get it all just right intensifies.

It isn't easy to wade through, especially for type-A people pleasers who want to do their best. And I know because I've experienced these pressures myself. My approach has changed through the years, and I hope that by sharing some of my story, I can help you avoid a restrictive mindset and embrace one that honors your body's needs. Planning what you'll eat and drink during a race is important, too, and we'll also go over that in this chapter. But take it from registered dietitian and Olympic Marathon Trials qualifier Starla Garcia—none of that matters if you don't have a solid foundation of healthy eating. (More background on Starla can be found in her athlete profile later in this chapter on page 53.)

I started learning this lesson as a freshman at Shippensburg University. Like many new college students, the transition from home-cooked meals to the dining hall led to experimentation with foods and a few extra pounds. I was running well—one runner-up NCAA title and two victories—but I couldn't help but wonder whether my changing shape was weighing me down.

When I looked at photos of distance-running pros, the women I aspired to be like, I homed in on their lean muscles. I figured that if I wanted to run like them, I needed to look like them. What I knew at the time was that weight was about calories in, calories out. So I tightened up, running more and eating less.

The weight came off, but it wasn't the only thing I'd lose. I'd always prided myself on running negative splits and kicking to the finish in races. At the Penn Relays my sophomore year, I tried to find that higher gear to close—and failed. I still won the 3K race but only because I'd led from the gun and managed to stay out in front of the pack. My lack of strength and power shook me; I just didn't feel like myself.

Soon, I stopped getting my period, and before long, my body began crumbling. I had stress fractures in my cuneiform, metatarsal, and fibula and annoying bouts of tendinitis. Until then, I'd convinced myself I remained in complete control, that my behaviors were normal for elite runners. But with those red flags, I began to see that my approach was unhealthy and detrimental. I needed to change before I dug myself into a deeper hole.

Fortunately, I had a strong support system and access to professionals, such as nutritionists, gynecologists, endocrinologists, and psychologists. With their help, I pulled back from the brink and began building the healthier, sustainable habits that would save my career. First, I had to adjust my mindset. No longer would I engage in a competition between me and the scale. Instead, I recommitted to running my best.

From there, I gained weight and got my period back; surprisingly, I learned that one reason I'd lost it was an elevated level of the hormone prolactin, which was caused by the irritation from my sports bras! I needed medication to get that level to drop and, thus, to resume my cycle. The journey wasn't an easy one, but I'm grateful I had that turning point at an early age. It gave me plenty of time to reset and build my body to withstand the demands of a pro career.

Contrast that with another major transition—when I came back after having Athens. The weight I had gained during my healthy pregnancy was far more than I'd ever put on in college. But all I'd learned through my career—including the two years I'd spent away from the sport—reinforced that rather than restriction, what I needed was a slow, natural path back toward higher-level running.

I stopped weighing myself, and instead of targeting a number, I aimed for a feeling—strong and smooth. I began working with a nutritionist who has a holistic approach. Together, we focused not on achieving a certain weight or body fat percentage but on improving my recovery. My process goals involved adding to my routine, not taking away from it. He challenged me to drink 90 to 100 ounces of water per day; increase both my carbohydrate and protein intake following hard sessions; and work flaxseed or chia seeds and their healthy omega-3 fatty acids into my diet, seven times a week.

This positive strategy paid off. Everything began coming together for me in the summer of 2020 when I was training for the Marathon Project coming up in December. I was back up to about 95 miles per week and running times in workouts I never had before—all while staying healthy, mind and body. Not only was I eating better before and after workouts, but I also found it easier than ever before to take in fluids and gels during long runs.

I felt like a final piece of the puzzle, one I'd still been fine-tuning in past marathons, was finally coming together. Less than a year after my first postpregnancy marathon, in which I qualified for the Olympic Marathon Trials, I felt primed for a personal best. This time, I knew I was going about it the right way; in fact, my lifestyle was so healthy and sustainable that I accidentally got pregnant with Rome during that period of intense training! So while I haven't had the chance to put all this newfound knowledge to the test during a race, I now have an even deeper trust in my body and its ability to perform, repair, and recover given the right resources.

HOW MUCH TO EAT

Myths and misinformation about food abound, and much of the general advice you hear doesn't consider the goals and lifestyle of a dedicated runner.

Most athletes can benefit from learning more about their individual needs, so if you're chasing a big goal, it's a great time to consult with a registered dietitian or qualified nutrition consultant. Look for someone who has experience with and certifications in working with athletes, for example, someone who's certified through the Academy of Nutrition and Dietetics as a Certified Specialist in Sports Dietetics (CSSD). But here, with the help of a few of those experts, we'll go over some of the basics.

First and foremost, you have to eat enough to support your training. You're aiming for energy balance—taking in sufficient fuel to cover everything you're expending while running, momming, working, playing, and just all around living as a human. Take in too little or burn too much, and you risk what's called low energy availability, or LEA (Melin et al. 2019).

A few years ago, experts at the Academy of Nutrition and Dietetics, Dietitians of Canada, and American College of Sports Medicine joined together to put out a statement on nutrition and athletic performance (Thomas, Erdman, and Burke 2016). Energy balance serves as "the cornerstone of the athlete's diet," they said, noting that it does the following:

- Offers more opportunities to get adequate macronutrients (carbohydrate, protein, and fat) and micronutrients (vitamins and minerals such as iron, vitamin D, and magnesium)

- Allows all your organs and systems to function properly
- Provides a solid baseline for your training and race-day fueling
- Protects you from long-term damage to your physical and mental health

Energy needs vary widely from runner to runner and change over time based on everything from your training to your hormonal cycle to how much you move around during the day. Even your stress levels, altitude, and the temperature outside play a role! So there's no one-size-fits-all solution, and commercial calorie-counting or food-tracking apps can be misleading and downright dangerous. Instead, tune in to your own cues of hunger, fullness, mood, and how well you run and recover.

Following are some signs that you may not be eating enough:

- Dragging on your runs or taking longer to recover afterward
- Constantly getting injured or sick
- Trouble concentrating
- Low mood or irritability (hanger, anyone?)
- General fatigue
- Irregular periods (more on this in chapter 5, on page 57)

If you notice them, you can course-correct before you experience some of the longer-term effects, including low bone density and fractures, heart damage, a sluggish metabolism, and fertility problems. Together, the constellation of harms caused by LEA is called relative energy deficiency in sport (RED-S). Not only can RED-S set you back in your running, but it can seriously harm your health.

In some cases, LEA or RED-S can be unintentional, the result of simply not knowing how to fuel properly. But in other instances, runners can develop disordered eating or eating disorders, including anorexia and bulimia. These can be life threatening and, sadly, are all too common in our sport—in one study, almost half of the women competing in sports that emphasize being lean, including long-distance running, were found to be at risk of eating disorders (Kong and Harris 2015).

In addition to the signs of RED-S, according to the National Eating Disorders Association (NEDA 2021), warning signs of eating disorders include a preoccupation with weight and food, skipping meals, frequently checking your body in the mirror, withdrawing from friends and family, and refusing to eat certain foods or food groups. If you start to feel like you're slipping toward these behaviors, it's important to get help quickly to protect your physical and mental health and, thus, help you to continue running strong. Reach out to a dietitian or a sport psychologist with experience in disordered eating. If you're in a crisis, call the NEDA Helpline at (800) 931-2237 or text "NEDA" to 741741.

WHAT TO EAT

So where should all that nourishing fuel come from? Again, there's no one eating plan that works for all runners. That's one of many reasons to think twice about fad diets, such as ketogenic and paleo, which claim to have the singular solution to better health and performance yet advocate cutting out whole food groups. Even diets that have to do with timing, rather than restricting food types, such as intermittent fasting, are often detrimental to women's hormonal systems—or haven't been studied in women at all (Roche 2020).

So while we can't give you hard and fast rules about a specific diet to follow, we can offer a few basic principles to guide you in creating a plan that's healthy and sustainable for you.

The United States Olympic & Paralympic Committee's sports nutrition team created three diagrams of the Athlete's Plate for easy, moderate, and hard days of training. They're a useful visual guide for your meals, especially with a small tweak from Maddie Alm, MS, RD, who's also an elite runner and a two-time U.S. Championships qualifier. She breaks the sections of the plate down into three main components:

- *Carbohydrate.* This is your body's primary source of fuel for aerobic activity, and your body stores it as glycogen to fuel your runs. It's also your brain's preferred energy source. Fill this part of your plate with whole grains, potatoes, or legumes.
- *Protein.* Best known for building muscle, protein also repairs and restores other tissues, including tendons and ligaments. It's critical for immune health too. Here, think poultry; fish; eggs; beef; and soy foods, such as tofu or tempeh.
- *Color.* Greens are good, but don't forget the reds, yellows, and purples too! Eating fruits and vegetables in all hues of the rainbow means you'll absorb all the micronutrients—vitamins and minerals—you need for healthy bones and blood. They also contain phytonutrients that regulate your body's inflammatory response. From arugula to eggplants to tomatoes, think about eating a rainbow of produce.

Top off each meal with a source of fat, which acts as a backup fuel source for easier runs, supports hormone health, and helps your body absorb many vitamins and minerals (Vitale and Getzin 2019). Polyunsaturated fat and monounsaturated fat—the kind found in avocados, nuts, flaxseed, chia seeds, and fatty fish such as salmon—best support heart and brain health (Gordon 2019).

These general guidelines can give you a starting point for portioning out your plate. From there, you can adjust by noticing how your body responds to specific foods and combinations. If you're feeling sluggish and low on energy, you probably need more carbohydrate. Struggling to recover from hard workouts? Prioritize protein. And make notes in your training log about any foods that leave you feeling particularly great (or awful).

We'll get into this even more in chapter 5, but the changes that come with your monthly cycle can also make a difference in how you respond to certain foods. So logging your period can also help you fine-tune your nutrition.

Most sports nutrition experts advocate getting as many of your nutrients as possible from whole foods, including fruits; vegetables; whole grains; dairy; and protein, such as beef, fish, and tofu or tempeh. I generally find I feel and perform better, especially as race day nears, when I eat more of these wholesome ingredients and fewer that are fried, high in refined sugar, or packaged and processed. But that doesn't mean these foods are "bad" or off limits. Dietitians such as Garcia also advocate an all-foods-fit philosophy—one that allows room for joy, culture, tradition, and pleasure en route to creating a sustainable plan that works for you.

Finally, there are times and situations when women have unique dietary needs. For instance, when you're pregnant or breastfeeding, you need more calories and a higher dose of certain nutrients (there's a bit more on that in chapter 6, on page 81). Also, although fad diets typically aren't the best for runners, you may have times when you're following a specific eating plan for health or personal reasons. This can include eating vegetarian or vegan for moral or religious reasons or going gluten free if you have celiac disease.

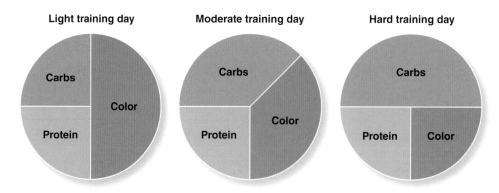

Athlete's Plates, for light, moderate, and hard days of training

In these instances, it's very important to pay attention to not only how much you're eating overall but also some of the micronutrients you're consuming. It's far easier to fall short when your diet has limits. So while dietitians and sports nutrition consultants can help you anytime, it's even more critical to book a visit with one if you're in one of these situations.

PROTEIN POWER

As mentioned, distance runners need lots of protein to repair their bodies from all that pounding—something I find it takes a conscious effort to consume. What makes it even more difficult is that your body absorbs protein better when it's spread throughout the day, versus lumped mainly into one or two big meals (Schoenfeld and Aragon 2018).

Along with ounces of water, protein is one of the only things you might want to count or track, just to ensure you're hitting the mark in terms of quantity and timing. I aim for about 15 to 30 grams, five times per day—three meals and two snacks—and find that's a good place for many other runners to start too. Here are some of my favorite ways to fit it in.

Snacks

These can be the toughest to tackle; go-to snacks such as cheese and nuts are a great start but usually won't get you all the way to 15 grams. Protein bars can work in a pinch, but I prefer less-processed options when possible. I like pickled eggs, cottage cheese, homemade protein energy balls with protein and collagen powder, smoked salmon, or a smoothie (see recipe later).

Breakfast

My go-to is plain Greek yogurt with fun fixings and flavors, such as nuts, chia seeds, Kashi cereal, pureed pumpkin and spices, blueberries, granola, or dried coconut—the combinations are endless! Other options include protein pancake mix, Dave's Bagels (which have 11 grams of protein), or eggs.

Lunch

I try to cook extra protein in advance so I have plenty of options to quickly add to salads and wraps through the week. Chicken, tempeh, hard boiled eggs, and canned chickpeas are easy to add to any meal.

Dinner

Most people naturally include protein in their evening meal. Elevate your game further by turning to sources with added nutritional value. Think wild-caught salmon, which has more vitamin D and omega-3 fatty acids than farmed (check out the salmon cakes recipe on page 47 for one great option); soup made with bone broth, rich in collagen and amino acids; or grass-fed beef, which contains an optimal balance of fatty acids as well as cancer-fighting antioxidants (Daley et al. 2010).

RECIPES

From my kitchen to yours, here are a few of my favorite nutrient-rich recipes to sustain your running.

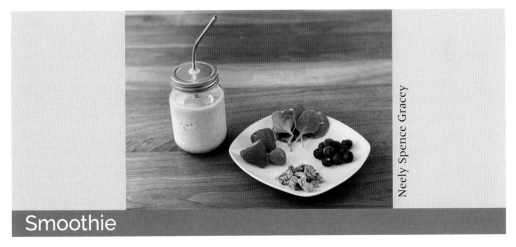

Neely Spence Gracey

Smoothie

This smoothie is easy, quick, and full of vitamins, protein, and anti-inflammatory omega-3 fatty acids to refuel and restore your body after a hard run.

- 1/2 frozen banana*
- 3/4 cup almond milk (or any milk)
- 4-6 ice cubes
- 1 tablespoon whole flaxseed or chia seeds
- 1 scoop of your favorite protein powder
- 1 scoop of collagen powder (optional)

Coaching: Blend all ingredients and enjoy.

*Feel free to add in berries or spinach for color and added nutrients.

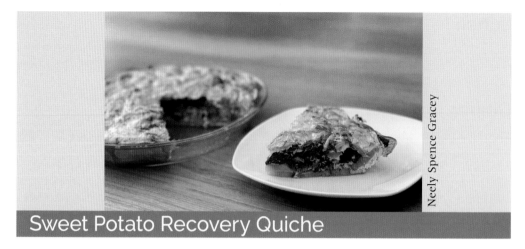

Neely Spence Gracey

Sweet Potato Recovery Quiche

This delicious meal is great for any time of day. It's protein packed and full of iron, vitamins, and calcium to boost your postworkout restoration.

Ingredients

- 1 large sweet potato (or 2 smaller ones) sliced very thin, peel only if desired
- 8 oz chopped and sautéed mushrooms (or substitute another sautéed veggie*)
- 1 small onion or 1/2 large onion, diced
- 1 bag (5 oz) fresh spinach, wilted
- 5 eggs
- 1/4 cup milk (or milk alternative)
- 1/4 cup plain Greek yogurt
- 1/4 teaspoon red pepper
- Salt and pepper to taste
- 1/2 cup shredded cheese divided in half

Coaching: Preheat the oven to 350 degrees. Thinly slice sweet potatoes and place in an oiled pie or eight-by-eight baking dish. Arrange to cover the whole bottom and sides. Spray with olive oil, then bake for 20 minutes. Meanwhile, heat a large skillet to medium high. Sauté mushrooms and onion for five minutes. Add in spinach, cover, and turn off heat (make sure spinach wilts sufficiently). In a bowl, combine all the other ingredients and half the cheese. Add in the cooked mushrooms and spinach. Pour the egg mixture into the baked sweet potato dish. Sprinkle remaining cheese on top, turn the oven up to 375 degrees, place on a cookie sheet, and bake for 45 minutes. Let stand a few minutes to cool before serving. Keeps and reheats well for meal prep.

*Bonus: You can add in other veggies or meat to your liking!

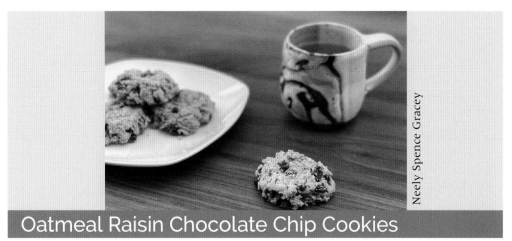

Neely Spence Gracey

Oatmeal Raisin Chocolate Chip Cookies

Wholesome and delish, these cookies won't disappoint. They're easy to whip up, and the spices, oats, and chocolate hit the spot after a good run (or really, anytime!).

Wet Ingredients

- 1 egg or flax egg*
- 1/4 cup melted coconut oil or softened butter
- 1/4 cup maple syrup
- 1 teaspoon vanilla

Dry Ingredients

- 1 1/4 cup almond flour or unbleached flour**
- 3/4 cup old-fashioned oats
- 1/2 teaspoon cinnamon
- 1/2 teaspoon baking powder
- 1/2 teaspoon baking soda
- 1/2 teaspoon salt

Yummy Ingredients

- 1/4 cup chocolate chips
- 1/4 cup raisins (or skip raisins, and add nuts or more chocolate chips if desired)

Coaching: Combine egg (or flax egg), coconut oil (or butter), maple syrup, and vanilla. Stir until smooth. Mix the rest of the ingredients in another bowl, then add to the wet mix. Stir until combined. Add in the chocolate chips and raisins. Scoop with a spoon into mounds. Bake at 350 degrees for 10 to 12 minutes on parchment paper. Yields 12 small cookies or 8 large.

*Flax egg: For a vegan option, combine one tablespoon ground flax mixed with three tablespoons water and let rest five minutes before adding to ingredients.
**For altitude baking, decrease flour from 1 1/4 cup to 1 cup instead.

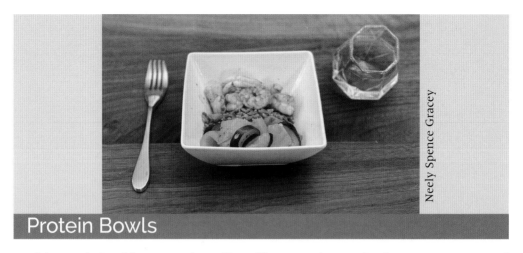

Neely Spence Gracey

Protein Bowls

This protein bowl has so much to offer—fiber, protein, veggies, immune support, and branched-chain amino acids for rebuilding fatigued muscles. The best part is that if you keep the staples around, it's a snap to build one anytime!

- Base (Choose one and cook one cup per its instructions.)
  - Quinoa (a gluten-free seed with protein)
  - Rice (Choose organic if you can to avoid arsenic residue.)
  - Farro (an ancient grain that provides even more fiber, minerals, and antioxidants than rice)
  - Bulgur wheat (a Mediterranean whole grain high in magnesium and iron)
  - Cauliflower rice (a nongrain option for low-mileage periods of training)
  - Couscous
- Protein (Choose one and cook 1 cup or 8 oz per instructions.)
  - Lentils
  - Beans
  - Chicken or shrimp
  - Steak
  - Tempeh or tofu
- Veggies (Make a combo of the following options and use what you have and what you like.)
  - Bell peppers
  - Onion
  - Mushrooms
  - Spinach
  - Kale
  - Broccoli
  - Cauliflower
  - Asparagus
  - Snap peas
  - Carrots
- 1 garlic clove
- Fresh ginger root (Peel and freeze the root, then finely grate or zest 1/4 inch of ginger root into the recipe.)
- 2 tablespoons of Bragg Liquid Aminos or soy sauce
- Sauce of choice: goddess dressing, peanut or teriyaki sauce from a bottle, or any homemade version

Coaching: Cook both base and protein per their instructions. Chop and sauté the veggies in a little olive oil. Add in the minced garlic, ginger, and Braggs. Stir to combine and cook until fragrant. Scoop the base and protein into a bowl and add the veggies and sauce on top.

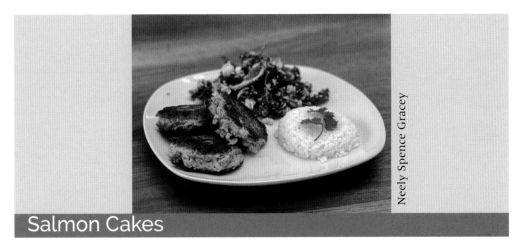

Neely Spence Gracey

Salmon Cakes

The key here is the wild-caught salmon, which contains more minerals, nutrients, vitamin D, protein, and healthy fat than other varieties. Farmed salmon, while cheaper, comes with more saturated fat, which is less ideal when you're asking your body and heart to perform athletically. You'll find really great flavor in this quick and easy recipe.

- 2 6 oz cans of wild-caught salmon
- 2 flax eggs (2 tablespoons ground flaxseed + 6 tablespoons water; let rest 5 minutes) or regular eggs
- 4 tablespoons almond meal or breadcrumbs
- 1/2 small onion or 1/4 large onion, diced
- 1/2 inch fresh, finely grated ginger (Hint: Buy a ginger root and freeze it; frozen, it keeps for a long time and is easier to grate. You can also use 1 tablespoon of dried ginger if necessary.)
- 1/4 cup fresh cilantro or parsley leaves, chopped
- 1/4 teaspoon crushed red pepper flakes
- 1/2 lime, juiced
- 1 teaspoon sesame oil
- Salt and pepper to taste

Coaching: Make the flax egg and let it sit five minutes while you prep the other ingredients. Add in the remaining ingredients and stir well. Shape the salmon cakes into eight small or five large patties. Heat four tablespoons of extra virgin olive oil (it's important to use extra virgin for higher-heat cooking) or avocado oil in a large saucepan over medium-high heat for one minute, then add the patties. Cook for three to five minutes, then flip. Cook for another two to four minutes. (They're also great in the air fryer—you can cook them for 12 minutes at 350 degrees for five patties or slightly less time if you divide them into eight.) Serve with a nice salad, sweet potato fries, rice, or any other side that strikes your fancy.

MIND YOUR MICROS

Even with a well-rounded diet, there are a few key vitamins and minerals runners are more likely to fall short on. To check your levels, you can work with a dietitian, a doctor, or a service such as InsideTracker, which allows you to order blood tests without a prescription. These nutrients include the following.

Iron

This mineral is critical to producing hemoglobin and myoglobin, proteins that infuse your muscles with energizing oxygen. We women are more likely to run low, in part, because we shed iron through menstrual blood. Iron-deficient runners might feel fatigued and low in motivation and eventually develop a condition called anemia. You can find it in beef, turkey, oysters, spinach, and fortified foods such as cereals (National Institutes of Health n.d.a.). Make sure to ask your doctor to test your ferritin levels and not just your iron levels—this measures the iron stored in your tissues. While experts debate the optimal level for athletes, my experience is that readings of less than 50 are on the low side, especially if you're training hard for your breakthrough.

Vitamin D

Any runner who lives north of Tennessee runs the risk of being deficient in the so-called sunshine vitamin. Ample amounts ensure bone health, decrease inflammation, help you sleep better, and improve communication between your muscles and your brain. You can find it in fatty fish, egg yolks, fortified foods, and mushrooms; your skin also produces vitamin D when exposed to sunshine (Gao et al. 2018; Thomas et al. 2016).

Magnesium

Nerves, muscles, and blood vessels rely on this electrolyte to function properly, and low levels can disrupt your sleep. You can find it in beans, nuts, seeds, spinach, and dairy foods (National Institutes of Health n.d.b.).

Vitamin B_{12}

If you eat a vegetarian, vegan, or plant-based diet, it's sometimes tough to get enough of this nutrient, which also plays a key role in the formation of red blood cells. You can find it in meat, eggs, or dairy foods (Klemm 2021).

Your dietitian or health care provider can advise you on how to boost low levels, including when to take a supplement and how to find a high-quality brand. Ideal ranges of these nutrients for athletes are different from those for the general population, so make sure your provider understands your lifestyle (and preferably, has experience working with endurance athletes). That's another benefit of services such as InsideTracker, which provide appropriate reference levels for a runner's lifestyle.

WHEN TO EAT

The final key component of a runner's diet is timing it all correctly. Energy imbalances can pop up hour by hour, messing with your mindset and ability to train well. About three meals and three snacks usually work for me, but if I'm hungry, I'll eat more! Your main goal should be to consume about the right amount throughout the day so that you're never famished or past satisfied.

Pay special attention to these key times:

- *Before a run.* Even if you run first thing in the morning, get at least a quick carbohydrate-rich snack. While some coaches recommend depleted runs to increase the body's fat-burning capacity, I find this strategy risky and counterproductive, especially for women. Running on empty can increase your injury risk, knock your hormone levels out of whack, and generally leave you feeling exhausted and low in confidence (Roche 2020).

- *During a run.* We'll delve into the details following, but in brief, any efforts lasting over 90 minutes could benefit from mid-run fueling. You know that feeling when you're dragging at the end of a long run? Getting ahead of it with fuel can keep you going strong until the end. Simple carbohydrate from gels, electrolyte drinks with calories, chews, or even real foods such as dried fruit or sweet potatoes provides instant energy. You'll also want to replenish fluids with 12 to 20 ounces of water per hour.

- *After a run.* Within an hour after you stop, aim for a snack with protein and carbohydrate to begin replenishing your glycogen stores and jump-starting the recovery process. This is one time when your hunger cues may mislead you; your appetite may be temporarily suppressed following a hard effort. Smoothies and shakes are your friends here if you can't stomach solid foods. If you skip this step, not only might you impair your recovery, but also your hunger will likely return with a rage later on.

DON'T FORGET TO DRINK

Hydration is another critical concern for runners. Ample fluids—and specifically water—keep oxygen-rich blood flowing through your veins, flush waste from your system, and keep your temperature regulated through sweating.

My rule of thumb for hydration is to take half your body weight in pounds, then add 15 to 20. That's the minimum of ounces of fluids I recommend that my athletes aim for in a day. I find it helpful to use a marked water bottle so I know how much I'm getting and how often I need to refill it (my favorite comes from 64Hydro—it marks off ounces by the hour and comes in all kinds of fun designs).

Sweat also depletes your stores of electrolytes, which are micronutrients, such as sodium, potassium, and magnesium, that are essential for muscle contraction and cardiovascular function. You can replenish these through food, but electrolyte-enhanced beverages can help too. During normal training, I swap about one daily bottle of water for a drink such as Sword, Honey Stinger, or Liquid I.V.

THE BUZZ ON CAFFEINE

Of course, there's one other frequently consumed beverage that might help your performance—coffee or any other drink, food, pill, or supplement containing caffeine. In study after study, caffeine has been shown to improve endurance in addition to its benefits for alertness, attention, and keeping your digestive system moving quickly when you need it most. According to the International Society of Sports Nutrition, the optimal timing is about 60 minutes before your run (Guest et al. 2021), but everyone reacts differently to the drug. You'll want to experiment with timing in training so you know what works for you on race day. One caution is that if you're using multiple caffeinated products, check to make sure your overall intake doesn't exceed about 400 milligrams a day, or you'll risk serious side effects, especially to your heart (Ellis 2020).

INDULGE OR REFRAIN?

Some athletes with big goals think they have to dial in all the details, right from the start. Often, runners will try to cut out everything "extra" from their diets and social lives at the start of a training cycle, including alcohol, dessert, nights out, and other so-called indulgences.

I admire their commitment and agree that hard training might not go hand in hand with a nightly pint of ice cream and a bottle of wine. But an overly rigid approach increases your risk of underfueling and is unsustainable over the long term. Not everyone drinks or likes sweets, of course, but I recommend keeping just-for-fun foods, drinks, and experiences in your life regardless.

For example, during hard marathon training, I'll do long runs on Saturday mornings, then relax a bit afterward. Dillon and I might spend the afternoon at the zoo with Athens, complete with an ice-cream stop; that evening, I often pour an extra glass of wine or stay up a bit to lounge in the hot tub or watch movies. This gives me something to look forward to outside of running and keeps me connected to friends and family, and if I do want to cut back on these things to boost my focus in the few weeks before a race, I feel confident I can handle it.

Sure, training can sometimes feel like a grind, but these types of mini mental resets make it easier to enjoy the journey. Since we're never guaranteed the outcome we want, our running—and our lives—are so much more worthwhile when we relish the process of striving.

BANISHING THE BONK

After my collegiate wake-up call, the next big shift I made in my nutrition as a runner occurred when I stepped up in distance. Running the mile or the 5K didn't deplete my body's glycogen stores, so what I ate the night before or the morning of a big run or race didn't matter so much. As long as it didn't upset my stomach, I was fine.

But when my long runs started topping two hours and my race distances extended to half and full marathons, I realized that what I ate the day before and the day of my harder efforts made a big difference in having the stamina, strength, and power to complete them. And because the body can store only a limited amount of glycogen, efforts of longer than about 90 minutes demand mid-run fueling.

I quickly realized that every workout and long run gave me an incredible opportunity to practice what would work for me on race day. There's a lot that's out of our hands when the gun goes off, but homing in on what I did the night before and the day of—creating a structure and routine that I knew would work for me—removed one more source of stress on race day.

The process has involved plenty of trial and error. For a while, my go-to dinner was pizza, but when I traveled to races, it was hard to find exactly the right type. Some gels upset my stomach or gave me an instant side stitch. I tried diluting them in water, which worked well—except during the New York City Marathon, when cold weather froze the solids to the bottom of my bottles, leaving me low on energy by the end of the race. But with time, I've developed a formula that works for me.

Prep for Performance

No matter how long you're racing, what you eat beforehand can make a difference in how you feel on the course. And as with everything else, fine-tuning your routine in training can pay off big-time on race day.

Try your best to eat before workouts and long runs, even early in the morning. Simple carbohydrate-rich foods, such as bananas, toast, rice cakes, or dry cereal, often work well; some runners can tolerate oatmeal and nut butter. On race day, I recommend waking up at least three hours before the start of a race and eating a larger portion of these "safe" foods to fuel your efforts.

For race distances of a half marathon or longer, it's also important to take in fuel as you go because your muscles can store only a limited amount of glycogen. If you've never tried fueling your long-distance runs, you'll be amazed at how much stronger, more energized, and faster you feel and how much better you'll perform.

The best fuel for mid-run is typically a simple carbohydrate, such as a gel or chew, designed specifically for this purpose. I tell my runners to aim for at least 30 grams of carbohydrate per hour. Garcia recommends aiming even higher; some of her runners can take in 80 to 90 grams per hour.

Every runner's digestive system and preferences are different, so you'll want to experiment with different types of fuel to see what works best for you. Also, give yourself some time to adjust to eating on the run. Just like your muscles, your gut can become better trained with time!

Following are some of the fueling options:

- Energy gels from brands such as Honey Stinger, Gu, Gatorade, Hüma, Spring, Maurten, or UCAN
- Chews or blocks from similar companies
- Bars, such as those from Clif, Picky Bars, or PowerBar
- Real ingredients, including honey packets, maple syrup, or even dates or sweet potatoes
- Homemade products, such as the Energy Squeeze from Shalane Flanagan and Elyse Kopecky's *Run Fast. Cook Fast. Eat Slow.* (Flanagan and Kopecky 2018) and their Giddy-Up Energy Bites from *Run Fast. Eat Slow.* (Flanagan and Kopecky 2016) or Matcha Lemon Date Bites from Lottie Bildirici, @runningonveggies on Instagram

Keep in mind that the energy you ingest takes about 20 minutes to become available and longer if you use products such as Maurten or UCAN, which are designed to be slow releasing. You'll want to begin fueling early and frequently to stay ahead of fatigue.

Race-day hydration is critical, too, and it's something else you'll want to pay attention to in training. Aim for at least 12 to 20 ounces of fluids per hour—more if it's hot and humid or you're just thirstier.

If you plan to use aid stations on the course, keep in mind that cups don't provide that much. You'll need to drink frequently or grab a few at a time. Of course, you can also take a handheld bottle, belt, or vest. You can also use sports drinks to provide some or all of the carbohydrate and calories you need. A word to the wise—look up what brand and flavor will be provided on the course and practice with it or carry your own if you have a brand preference that won't be provided.

Practice Makes Perfect

Rehearsing all this—the types of foods and drinks, the logistics of consuming them on the move, and the timing of when you take them—is critically important for your race-day success. All runners have their quirks and preferences, but here are some ideas to start with as you plan your own strategy (see table 4.1). The more you experiment during training, the more confident you'll feel heading into race day.

Table 4.1   Prime to Peak

Timeframe	Try . . .	Neely's go-to
Taper week (or weeks)	Keep your diet and habits relatively consistent. You've been dialing in what works for you throughout training, so no need to mess with much now. Because most of your hard work is done, you can place less emphasis on protein and more on carbohydrate, making sure you have at least one or two good sources with every meal. Some runners switch to simpler, easier-to-digest carbohydrate a day or two before a race, which is fine.	I focus on getting complex carbohydrate, such as brown rice or whole-grain bread, for instance, adding garlic bread to my salad and granola to my yogurt. I also stop drinking alcohol and cut back on sugar and caffeine in the month before a race to improve sleep, reduce inflammation, and enhance hydration. This also gives me a psychological cue that race day is almost here; it's a lifestyle I know I can sustain for this short period.
Dinner the night before	Eat a meal with a source of lean protein and carbohydrate-rich foods. Think pasta, sweet potato, pizza, rice, or even sushi. Aim for options that will be easy to find before a race, and experiment to see what works best for your digestive system. Many runners find foods high in fiber or fat don't work as well, but again, your preference may vary.	I eat rice; steamed or grilled veggies; and chicken, prepared simply.
Hydration the day (or days) before	Starting three to four days out from race day—or the day before a long run or hard workout—alternate water and electrolyte-enhanced beverages.	I drink Sword, Cure, Liquid I.V., Nuun, Hydrant, or SOS. (Sword is my go-to for races.)
Fueling the morning of	Get up early enough to eat a meal you've practiced with, rich in simple carbohydrate, such as bananas, toast, rice cakes, or dry cereal or oatmeal and nut butter.	I eat Honey Stinger waffles, a banana, and Honey Stinger gummies.
Hydration the morning of	Start the day with a drink of water; drink water or an electrolyte beverage with your prerun meal.	On hot days and before races and long runs, I drink at least 10 ounces of Sword before heading out.
Fueling during (for long runs of at least 60 to 90 minutes and races of half-marathon or longer distance)	Aim for at least 30 grams and as many as 80 to 90 grams of carbohydrate per hour. Plan out your timing: consider eating a gel right before your start and topping off your stores at regular intervals.	I take a swig of Sword and a Maurten gel about five minutes before the start, then at least every 40 minutes throughout the race.
Hydration during a race	Drink at least 12 to 20 ounces of fluids per hour, either from aid stations, your own bottle or hydration system, or a combination of the two.	I wash my gels down with Sword from my bottles and grab a cup or two when I need water.

Rewriting the Rules: Starla Garcia

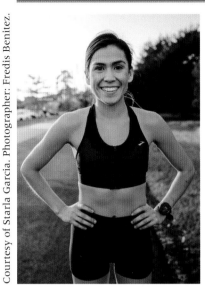

Starla Garcia is an Olympic Trials marathoner with a thriving business as a dietitian, one that combines intuitive eating, sports nutrition, and a focus on culture to help runners reach their goals. Her inspiration comes from her own struggles with food and eating—ones she shares openly in hopes of helping other runners overcome similar issues.

Beginning in high school, Starla began to absorb the message that if only she were thin enough, she'd be faster. On top of that, she felt a dissonance between her background as a Latina and the running world. Not only did she look different from most of her teammates and competitors, but also the messages she received about healthy eating ran counter to her heritage and traditions.

"I was being taught cultural foods cause obesity and heart disease and we need to limit them; we need to tell people to not have tortillas," she says. Even at the time, it didn't sit right: "This is my culture. And now I'm being taught that this is wrong. Why is that? Should I be limiting this so I can fit in as an athlete?"

She began restricting her eating, and by her sophomore year at the University of Houston, she'd developed anorexia with restriction. Her running began to suffer, and her health was in danger.

At the urging of her coach and with help from her teammates, Starla first sought treatment in 2009. Looking back, she sees that even at her lowest points, she had a desire to help others in a way that honored their identities and culture. "I always had this pull that when I entered recovery, this was the work I was going to be doing," she says. "That was a huge driving force in my own recovery process."

The summer after Starla graduated college in 2012, she committed to recovery. She also began to face and repair the extensive damage her eating disorder had caused. A DEXA scan informed her she had osteopenia, weakening of the bones, due to loss of a menstrual cycle and restriction of foods throughout her collegiate training. Healing was hard work, but as she pursued it, running transformed for her. Instead of a way to reshape her body, it became a method of exploring the world around her and herself. She practiced intuitive eating, following her cues of hunger, and reincorporated cultural foods, such as tamales and tortillas. "Instead of fighting my body every day, I was actually finally listening," she says.

As a result, she regained her natural glow; her Instagram handle @starla_shines and the name of her nutrition coaching practice, The Healthy Shine, came from a comment by a teammate about how her personality shone through again after recovery.

And her performances soared. At Grandma's Marathon in 2019, she ran 2:47:08, just over two minutes off the Olympic Marathon Trials qualifying standard—all while fueling properly, taking in 10 gels on the course. And at her hometown Houston Marathon in January 2020, she crossed the line in 2:43:56, qualifying her to line up for the Olympic Marathon Trials in Atlanta the next month.

To her, success on the road was about more than her own goals—she aimed to blaze a path forward for other women of color. And it gave her credibility as a dietitian. When runners seek her help with fueling, she can truly connect and help them break free of restrictive thinking.

Athletes often cringe when she tells them the maximum amount of carbohydrate they could ingest to improve their performance during marathons and other long races—up to 80 to 90 grams per hour. With patience, she helps them overcome deep-rooted dietary fears and build a healthy baseline of daily nutrition. That way, they can handle more fuel, both digestively and emotionally.

It's hard work—but so is training, she points out. Pursuing nutrition just as passionately as your workouts means you're not leaving anything on the table, figuratively or literally, in pursuit of being your best—and finding your own confident, healthy glow.

FROM BARRIER TO BREAKTHROUGH

Nutrition is a critical piece of success for runners, but when most people think of dialing it in, they first plan ways to restrict. I challenge you to set small goals to fuel better instead.

Barrier

Whenever my mileage ramps up, I feel like I'm dragging.

Breakthrough Goals

Choose one or more.

I will do the following:

- Eat more overall, especially before, during, and after long runs and workouts
- Check to see whether my plate matches up to the Athlete's Plate diagrams on page 42, and if not, see what portion I need to add to
- Be sure I am not going longer than three hours without eating and drinking

------

Barrier

I feel like I eat pretty well but really want to focus on improving my diet during this training cycle.

Breakthrough Goals

Choose one or more.

I will do the following:

- Make sure I'm getting 15 to 30 grams of protein at each meal and snack
- Calculate my daily fluid needs and aim to meet them
- Add in another color of fruits or veggies to one meal per day
- Make an appointment with a dietitian or sports nutrition consultant for personalized advice

------

Barrier

I have major gut problems fueling during a race.

Breakthrough Goals

Choose one or more.

I will do the following:

- Consider whether I'm underfueling overall, which often exacerbates gut health issues
- Start slowly to train my gut, adding just one gel at a time and working my way up
- Try a wide variety of products—including sports drinks, instead of gels; slow-releasing products, such as Maurten or UCAN; or whole foods, such as dried fruit—until I find something that works for me
- Consult a dietitian or sports nutrition consultant for a personalized evaluation and plan

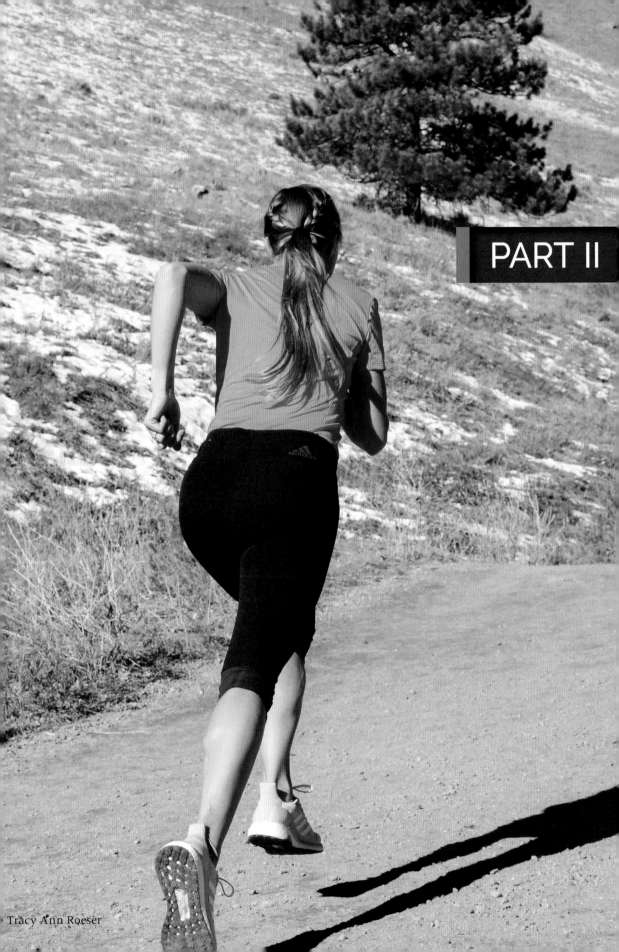

PART II

Tracy Ann Roeser

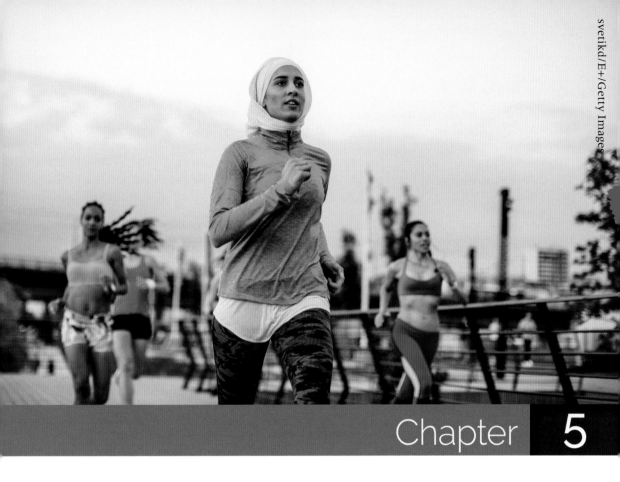

Chapter **5**

Master Your Cycle

" Celebrate the power of your body and what it's capable of. Recognize and embrace your own unique strengths that make you unstoppable. "

Elise Cranny, Olympic 5,000-meter runner

In the words of exercise physiologist Dr. Stacy Sims, women are not small men. From monthly hormone cycles to the pressures of the diet culture, female athletes have unique characteristics that influence their health and performance.

Fortunately, coaches and athletes have begun openly discussing topics that were once taboo, from periods to negative body image. Experts like Dr. Sims now study women in the lab and use the results to share practical guidance. And technological tools, such as apps to track your menstrual cycle, make it easier than ever to work with your physiology, not against it. Add it all up, and as female runners we have more power than ever before to reach our goals in a healthy, sustainable way.

GOING WITH THE FLOW

Everyone has bad race days, and from the start of the 2015 U.S. 20K Championships in New Haven, Connecticut, I struggled. My legs felt heavy and my breathing was ragged. As early as 5K, I was already near redlining, far outside my comfort zone.

The whole race, I focused on following the pack. *Don't let them get away from you*, I thought. *Hold on as long as you can.* Beginning at the halfway mark, I'd hoped to start picking up the pace. But as each mile clicked by, my body let me know that it wasn't ready to accelerate. Instead, I simply hung on for dear life.

Finally, with about two and half miles to go, two other runners and I—Ali Williams and Blake Russell—entered a quiet, tree-lined section of the course, leading into a downhill. *Now's my chance.* I knew I was strong on descents and that Ali, a former 1,500-meter runner, had a powerful kick. *It's now or never if I want to break away.*

My eyes locked on a purple kit ahead—Brianne Nelson, another runner I'd frequently competed against this year. I harnessed every last bit of energy and managed to slightly speed up, hold off Blake and Ali, and finish fourth in 1:08:02. But I couldn't catch Brianne, who finished third and more than 30 seconds in front of me, and the effort felt more challenging than I thought it should have.

I was proud of myself for sticking with it on a tough day when I had nothing more to give. Still, I knew the result didn't reflect my hard work in training or my current fitness level.

Fast-forward to the next month at the USATF 10 Mile Championships, held in Minneapolis–St. Paul, Minnesota, on October 4. From the start, I felt strong, calm, and confident. I put the last race out of my mind and focused on the positive. *Someone has to win today—why not me?* I thought.

With two miles to go, I was running in a pack with Brianne as well as Alexi Pappas and Laura Thweatt. This time, I had no hesitation about making a move. Relaxed, controlled, and focused, I put in a strong surge for a full half mile. My next split was a 5:12 mile—on an uphill! This time, when I asked my body to give more, it responded with a resounding yes.

Olympian Molly Huddle (you read about her on page 34) had led from the gun and was out of my reach—in fact, she'd dominated the whole season and set a new course record of 51:44 that day. Still, I steadily gained ground, closing with a 4:59 mile and placing second in 53:03. Short of claiming the win, it was everything I'd imagine a perfect race to be.

The difference in how I felt was remarkable. The first race was all about survival, whereas the second was a career highlight. Sure, I'd done a couple of good workouts in between. The main difference? Where I was in my menstrual cycle. The 20K race fell the week before my period, whereas at the 10 mile, I had just started it.

Many women dread racing during their periods. Some even use birth-control pills to tinker with the timing. To some extent, I understand this urge. As I mentioned in chapter 4, I had amenorrhea—aka absence of a period—in college. When I regained it, my cycle wasn't completely regular yet. Whether my races were three or six weeks apart, I almost always seemed to get my period right before. I worried about tampon strings popping out of my tiny buns and, depending on the color of my sponsor kits, visible leaks.

But after spending five years fighting to have a period at all, I wasn't about to wish it away. Once I began marking the day it started in my training log, I saw that despite some minor inconveniences, it was actually a critical advantage.

During my period and the week that followed, I could knock hard runs out of the park and crush the final miles of tough races. The week before, I'd feel lousy during workouts and sometimes cut them short, doing an easier tempo run, adding in more recovery, or decreasing the number of repetitions. Afterward, I'd struggle to recover. All this, I'd come to learn, happened midway through my luteal phase, halfway between ovulation and my period.

Eventually, I began to hope I'd get my period right before a race. This mindset shift allowed me to think and train differently. Gradually, I learned to embrace the strength and power my hormones gave me. And while it started with awareness of my period, it opened the door to completely embracing all the gifts that make me, as a female athlete, unique.

HELLO, HORMONES

For years, exercise scientists studied only men; women's fluctuations might muck up the results of their experiments, they theorized. However, it's those very ebbs and flows that we as women need to understand to maximize our training and performance, as Dr. Sims explains in her influential 2016 book on the topic, *ROAR: How to Match Your Food and Fitness to Your Unique Female Physiology for Optimum Performance, Great Health, and a Strong, Lean Body for Life* (Sims and Yeager 2016).

For half of the average 28-day cycle, levels of the hormones estrogen and progesterone are low, and our physiology works most similarly to men's, Dr. Sims notes. But in the other half of the month, hormone levels rise after you ovulate in part to prepare your body for a potential pregnancy. During all or part of this time, you might notice some changes, she explains in *ROAR*. These changes include the following:

- Your body may use less glycogen and more fat for fuel, making high-intensity efforts more challenging.
- Your sweat response could be slower to turn on while your core temperature increases, leaving you prone to overheating.
- Your muscles may break down more quickly and repair more slowly, meaning you need longer to recover between efforts.
- Fluid often shifts into your cells, leaving you feeling bloated.
- Every effort might feel harder, thanks to increased fatigue in your central nervous system.

Your hormone levels tend to drop, alleviating these concerns, right around the time of your period. So it makes sense that I'd have my best races then, and I'm not alone. Elise Cranny also notices a performance boost when her period starts and for a few days after. And Paula Radcliffe ran 2:17:18 at the 2002 Chicago Marathon—a world record that stood until 2019—while coping with cramps (BBC Sport 2015).

Some of the athletes I coach have very different experiences. Many find that symptoms, such as heavy bleeding, gastrointestinal distress, or serious cramps, make training and racing more difficult on their periods; others get migraines and can't run at all during certain phases of their cycles. Disrupted sleep, which often happens right before your period, can also affect your ability to recover.

Scientists are now doing their best to explore the effects of the menstrual cycle on performance. On average, studies show that factors such as $\dot{V}O_2max$ (Rael et al. 2021) and lactate threshold (Dean et al. 2003)—key variables that go into doing well in endurance events—don't shift by phase. However, that doesn't tell the story of what happens in your own body. Just as Elise and I and the athletes I coach notice changes by phase, you might too. But as I experienced during the 20K Championships, no matter what, you can still finish strong and feel proud of your efforts.

TRACKING YOUR CYCLE

Fortunately, thanks to technology, there are more tools than ever to help you monitor your menses. First, here are a few basics: An average cycle is 28 days, but the typical range is from 24 to 38 days (Office on Women's Health n.d.). Your period might come like clockwork or fluctuate from month to month. You're least likely to have regular cycles soon after you start getting your periods and then again in your 40s as your body gets closer to menopause.

You can keep tabs on all this by simply marking the dates of your period in your training log (I write mine in my trusty *Believe Training Journal*). My coaching clients will often include this information in the "post workout notes" in their electronic training logs on Final Surge. You can also use a period-tracking app. FitrWoman and Wild AI are geared specifically toward athletes and pair information about where you are in your cycle with tips about training and nutrition strategies to maximize it; you can also track your period in Garmin Connect if that's the brand of GPS watch you use.

Most experts recommend tracking for at least three months. That way, you'll have a better idea of whether any trends you see are repeated over time.

I found this approach particularly helpful after having Athens. Every effect of my cycle—from the dips in energy and headaches I felt before my period to the performance boost after I got it—felt more intense after I stopped breastfeeding and resumed menstruating. Using the app gave me a better handle on where I was and what to expect so I could make changes to my strategy as needed. Tracking can also help you pinpoint when you're entering perimenopause or have completed the menopausal transition (which you can read more about below).

If you have a coach, I urge you to find a comfortable way to share this information. I know it isn't always easy to bring up. After all, when I got my very first period in eighth grade, I couldn't bring myself to tell my coach—who was also my dad! Midway through a run soon afterward, he nonchalantly said, "So your mom said you got your period." I wanted to die of embarrassment, but he was calm and collected, asking me to let him know if it ever interfered with my running.

We've all come a long way since then. Digital logs allow you to transmit the details just like you would any other data; FitrWoman has a companion app, FitrCoach, which enables seamless communication. Regardless of how you share, there are many good reasons to speak freely. The more we discuss these topics, the more easily any remaining stigma will fade away.

THE BIG TRANSITION

Now you're starting to see how shifting hormones can change how you feel, sleep, and respond to training within the month during your cycle. Around the time you become a masters runner—age 40 and older—you might notice even wider swings.

As your reproductive years draw to a close, your estrogen and progesterone levels decline more precipitously (Kuzma 2020). Your periods will start to become more irregular, and symptoms, such as hot flashes and sleep problems, begin to set in. Congratulations! You're in perimenopause, the official transition time before your cycle stops altogether.

If you're in the middle of this transition, you're not alone—and once again, though women in this phase were previously ignored in exercise science labs, researchers and athletes are now stepping up to help us all better understand and navigate it.

Most women have their final periods between 40 and 58 years old, and perimenopause can begin about four to eight years earlier (North American Menopause Society n.d.). So you might notice wonky periods and other signs as early as your 30s (Mayo Clinic 2021b). Hormonal shifts during perimenopause and menopause can affect your running in several ways, but fortunately, there are ways to offset the negative effects.

- *Cool down.* Lower estrogen levels affect your body's thermostat, which is in the brain region called the hypothalamus. Not only does this cause hot flashes and night sweats, but you might also find that you have more difficulty training in hot weather. The good news is that exercising regularly may reduce the number of hot flashes you have in the first place (Stojanovska et al. 2014). To beat the heat on runs, Dr. Sims recommends a dose of the amino acid beta-alanine beforehand to help open up your blood vessels and improve your body's self-cooling system. You can also time your runs for cooler parts of the day, decrease your core temperature by sipping ice-cold water or a slushie, remove extra layers, or add an ice vest or chilled bandana.

- *Sleep soundly.* You'll also produce less of the hormone melatonin, which promotes sleep in part by lowering your core temperature (Society for Endocrinology 2018). To get a better and more rejuvenating night's rest, boost your levels by drinking tart cherry juice before bed, and soak up night sweats with moisture-wicking sleepwear and sheets.

- *Power up.* Hormonal shifts mean it's harder to build and maintain muscle and your percentage of fast-twitch muscle fibers declines. Dr. Sims says adding in more strength training; plyometrics; hills; and short, fast intervals can strengthen muscles and bones while improving your neuromuscular connections—the communication between brain and body that enables you to recruit muscle fibers quickly and efficiently. Just make sure you listen to your body and add in more rest days, too, to recover from all that hard work; it might take you a little longer to bounce back than it used to.

- *Fuel wisely.* Alterations in metabolism and nutrient absorption mean you could benefit from tweaks to your nutrition. Lower estrogen decreases your body's ability to use insulin to process glucose (Yan et al. 2019), so simple sugars don't always work as well to fuel your runs. Experiment with products that include some protein and fat, such as Spring or Hüma brand gels. Throughout the day, aim to cut added sugar and instead focus on getting more complex carbohydrate, high-quality protein (including that from yogurt and meat, which includes the amino acid leucine), healthy omega-3 fat from foods such as fish and walnuts, and foods rich in calcium and vitamin D to protect bone and heart health.

Many of the challenges linked to perimenopause and menopause are relatively short term, and once your period stops completely, you'll likely find yourself settling into a new normal. If you trained hard in your younger years, you might notice a more permanent slowdown from your previous best times. That said, if you started running later in life, there's no reason you can't continue to improve long into your masters career. And regardless of age and phase, you can always set big goals and work to be the best version of yourself.

USE IT, DON'T LOSE IT

While three months of tracking your period will give you useful data, I personally think the timing of your period is a valuable piece of information to have all the time. Of course, delayed or missing periods might mean you're pregnant. This can change your timeline surrounding goals, as I experienced in 2020! They might also indicate you're nearing menopause, which could require some tweaks to your routine. And as we touched on in chapter 4, irregularities in your cycle could also be a red flag that you're not striking the right balance between training, rest, and fueling or even that you might have other health problems.

In that way, menstruation is a huge gift of female physiology. Our magical, wonderful bodies work hard to keep everything in balance. When something's off, they begin shutting down less-essential functions—such as those that lead to reproduction—to protect the systems and structures we need to sustain life. That means we have an early warning sign that something's amiss.

In one recent study, female soccer players had an increased risk of injury if they were even a few days late for their period (Martin et al. 2021). The earlier you notice that you might be off track, the faster you can get back in control by adding recovery days, boosting your fuel intake, reducing or managing life stress, or potentially taking a few rest days. If you aren't sure where to start or have tried a few things and still have irregular bleeding, it's a good idea to check in with your primary care doctor, a sports medicine physician, an endocrinologist (a doctor who treats hormone problems), or a registered dietitian who specializes in working with athletes.

When I lost my period, I saw all these specialists. I was eventually diagnosed with hypothyroidism, a condition in which the thyroid gland is sluggish. For me, it's genetic; both my mom and her mom had it. Now, I take synthetic thyroid hormone to prevent long-term health complications, such as joint pain and heart disease. While it wasn't the cause of my amenorrhea, it was another piece of the hormone puzzle that came together only because I was paying attention to my period.

I might sound like a broken record, but I can't say it often enough: Losing your period is not a badge of honor or a normal consequence of hard training. It's your body's way of telling you something isn't right. Figuring out the cause—and correcting it—could not only power you to your breakthrough, but it could also protect your health for many more breakthroughs to come.

As the research evolves, keep tabs on the work of scientists such as Dr. Sims for the latest insights and advice. Her book on this topic, *Next Level: The Ultimate Guide to Keep Kicking Ass and Competing Through Menopause and Beyond*, is scheduled to be released in May 2022.

TWEAKS TO TRY

Because every woman's cycle affects her differently—based on everything from her genetics to her lifestyle—there's no one-size-fits-all recommendation for optimizing your training and nutrition at each phase. However, Dr. Sims and other scientists, nutrition experts, and coaches have come up with a variety of strategies that might benefit athletes. You can experiment with these and note the results in your training log, fine-tuning what makes you feel and perform your best.

Sideline PMS Symptoms

To reduce bothersome symptoms, such as cramps, bloating, and gastrointestinal distress, Dr. Sims recommends this protocol each night for a week before your period starts: 250 milligrams of magnesium, 45 milligrams of zinc, one baby aspirin (80 to 81 milligrams), and one gram of omega-3 fatty acids, such as flaxseed or fish oil. This combo suppresses the production of compounds called prostaglandins, which cause your uterus to contract and contribute to diarrhea and other GI issues.

Load Up on Leucine

Women always have a harder time building muscle than men, an effect that's heightened in your high-hormone phase, Dr. Sims says. She recommends women focus on protein containing the high-quality amino acid leucine, especially after exercise. You can find leucine in whey protein, Greek yogurt, salmon, lean beef, and preworkout blends containing branched-chain amino acids.

Cycle Your Seeds

Some nutrition experts recommend eating raw seeds at different parts of your cycle to balance out hormone levels. To do this, eat one tablespoon each of freshly ground flax and pumpkin seeds the first 13 to 14 days, and the second half, switch to one tablespoon each of ground sunflower and sesame seeds. I often blend my seeds into smoothies or sprinkle them on yogurt. Studies of this technique aren't conclusive, but because seeds have other health benefits and few risks, there's little harm in trying them (Healthline n.d.).

Outsmart Headaches

Personally, headaches are one of my biggest PMS complaints. I ward them off by putting extra focus on hydration, both with water and electrolyte drinks. On long runs during this time in my cycle, I've gone through more than 40 ounces of fluids when I might normally drink less than half of that. This also helps because high-hormone days often raise your core temperature, as Stacy writes in *ROAR*. She also recommends foods rich in nitric oxide—think beets, pomegranates, spinach, and watermelon—to dilate your blood vessels, relieving pressure in your skull.

Reduce Volume or Add Recovery

Again, just because running feels harder at one point in your cycle than another doesn't mean you have to throw in the towel. In fact, practicing your perseverance during training can give you confidence for racing well anytime. However, you might find you need more recovery after a hard workout during certain phases. If you're feeling more fatigued than usual, you can add in an extra easy run or a cross-training day. After I had Athens and the effects of my cycle hit harder, Dillon and I decided to start planning my training around my cycle ahead of time. I would purposely schedule a lighter week—perhaps with a shorter long run or a less intense workout—for that high-hormone phase, when I knew I'd feel the worst. That way, I didn't need as much recovery and felt ready to hit it hard again when my hormone levels stabilized. Overall, I just felt so much better and performed well as a result. I also structure training this way for many of the athletes I coach.

PICK YOUR PRODUCT

Like birth control, period products are highly personal and may take some trial and error to get just right. My biggest advice is to practice long runs using whatever type of protection you plan to race in. That way, you can troubleshoot issues, such as chafing, leaks, or pressure, and have one less thing to worry about on race day. The most common choices include the following.

ABOUT BIRTH CONTROL

Contraception is yet another consideration in this equation. Doctors once prescribed the pill to women with amenorrhea from training as a way of restoring their periods and protecting their bone health. That turned out to be a bad idea.

Most oral contraceptives involve three weeks of external hormones, then one week of inactive pills, during which time you'll get your period. But that type of bleed is a sign of withdrawal from the hormones—it's not the same as naturally getting your period—so it can mask underlying irregularities in your cycle.

Another problem is that unlike natural estrogen, which protects bone health, the way estrogen from pills is metabolized may weaken bones, especially in young women (Singhal et al. 2019). Oral contraceptives also have other side effects athletes should consider, including weight gain, low mood, and a greater risk for blood clots (Mayo Clinic 2021a).

Of course, pills do work well at preventing pregnancy provided you take them properly. They can also allow you to delay the timing of your period if you truly want to avoid getting it for a race, trip, or other event. However, it's important to note that taking pills means you can't use your period as a sign that you're in energy balance. You'll have to keep tabs on other symptoms—such as your mood or how well you're recovering after workouts—to make sure you're not underfueling or overtraining.

In fact, any type of hormonal birth control—including patches, implants, and vaginal rings—can influence your period. Tracking your cycle can still help you sync up how you typically feel and perform at various points along the way. However, you might notice the fluctuations don't have as large of an effect as they do for your friends who use different forms of contraception.

Many runners who aren't planning families in the near future use an intrauterine device, or IUD. Some, like the Mirena, release hormones. Others, like the Paragard, are made of copper and don't. In either case, they last years after insertion, are reversible once they're removed, and lack some of the common side effects of oral birth control. Some women have lighter periods with an IUD, and others have no periods at all, which can be great if you normally have super-heavy or painful periods. Note that like any form of birth control, they're not 100 percent effective—less than 1 in 100 women gets pregnant while using them (Centers for Disease Control and Prevention 2020), and I was one of them! But they're still a great option for many athletes.

In short, the form of birth control that's best for you is an individual decision you should make in consultation with your doctor, knowing the unique concerns runners face. Once you select a method, you'll want to keep that in mind when it comes to monitoring your cycle. This is another reason it's great to have a health care team—including a gynecologist—with experience treating athletes.

Tampons

Of course, they're widely available, relatively inexpensive, and easy to borrow from a running buddy or buy in a public bathroom if you forget them. You do have to replace them frequently to reduce the risk of complications, such as toxic shock syndrome (TSS) (Cleveland Clinic n.d.), and if you're a heavy bleeder, they can leak during long races. I also found chemicals in nonorganic tampons made my cramping worse.

Pads

No TSS risk here, but you might face bunching, rubbing, and chafing. For these reasons, many runners opt to go another route.

Menstrual Cups

These flexible receptacles are usually made of silicon and fit snugly around your cervix to catch blood as it leaves your uterus. Inserting them properly takes a little practice, but many women—myself included—find them comfortable, convenient, and leakproof. Brands such as Pixie Cup, DivaCup, or Lunette hold a lot more fluid than a tampon or pad and can usually be left in for 8 to 12 hours, giving you one less thing to worry about on race day (Kuzma 2015b).

Period Clothing

All-in-one absorbent bottoms by companies such as Thinx and Knix work well for women who are uncomfortable with wearing something internally. You can choose from a variety of styles, including everything from thong underwear to training shorts, capris, and leggings. They're also eco-friendly because you simply wash them after wearing.

RACE-DAY ARRANGEMENTS

By now, you've learned not to fear the flow. Your period doesn't have to be detrimental to your performance, but it pays to prepare for what to do if it coincides with race day.

Practice Beforehand

The "nothing new on race day" mantra applies here, big-time. Pay attention to how your period affects you during training and what steps make it less bothersome and more comfortable. Trying Dr. Sims' PMS supplement protocol (page 63), hydrating more, and reducing your training volume in your taper could mitigate any negative effects of racing during this part of your cycle. And if you try them in training, you'll have that much more confidence on race day.

Include Dress Rehearsals

Anytime you have your period during training, try running with the types of products you plan to race in. As I mentioned, I personally like menstrual cups—when you insert them right, you can't feel them at all, but the process does take a bit of practice. Period clothing, meanwhile, means you can skip an extra step of inserting a tampon or cup. However, you'll definitely want to find shorts or underwear with a comfortable fit for fast mileage.

Pack Your Bag

Whether you're using a cup, clothing, tampons, or another option, make sure you have everything you need—plus extras if possible—tucked into the gear you're taking to the race. Also, consider taking hand sanitizer if you're going to be inserting new items or handling used ones (now that we've all been through COVID, we know it's probably a good idea to bring that everywhere anyway).

Time It Right

Because a cup holds plenty of fluids and doesn't increase your risk of TSS, you can put it in on race morning and forget about it. If you're using tampons or pads, you'll want to change them as close to the start time as possible, especially for longer races, such as half and full marathons. Build this into your prerace routine (and scope out the portable toilet situation beforehand).

Ward It Off

There's one other option if you already take birth control pills—skipping the inactive pills to shift the timing of your period. Best to talk with your doctor about this one, though many say there's no harm in doing this every once in a while because being on the pill already manipulates your cycle (Kuzma 2015a).

RECLAIM YOUR BODY IMAGE

Success as a female athlete involves tuning in to your internal cues, the unique physiological characteristics that make your amazing, powerful body tick. Another benefit of this approach is that it drowns out some of the external noise that can stand in the way of success—messages from all around us about how we "should" look, fuel, or train. While we touched on this in chapter 4, I want to take a moment here to talk a little more about body image because it's such a difficult topic for women runners.

As a young athlete, I put an outsized focus on achieving a lean runner's physique. I judged my fitness based on the definition of my abs, my proximity to an arbitrary "race weight," and how my body compared to the bodies of my athletic idols and competitors. When I read over my running logs from those years, I wish I'd put all that energy into how I felt instead.

I cringe when I reflect on how I sometimes "didn't have time" to eat and how during my last prerace pit stop, I'd lift up my shirt in the bathroom mirror to make sure I could see my abs. As long as I looked fit, I thought, I was ready to compete! I was never diagnosed with an eating disorder, but I—like Elise Cranny, who's profiled at the end of this chapter—definitely restricted myself in ways that were unhealthy. That attitude stuns and saddens me now, and I wonder how much better I could've been if I hadn't been so caught up in appearances.

Now, I know the real keys to success as a distance runner—an engaged core, a strong posterior chain, and a well-developed aerobic system—aren't visible in the mirror. Your abs tell you more about your genetics than they reveal about your strength or your ability to close in the final stretch of a tough race. Women with a wide range of body types can—and do—climb podiums, claim medals and championships, and get the best out of themselves on the racecourse.

Meanwhile, placing all your energy on a number on the scale can lead you quickly down a rabbit hole of disordered or restricted eating; low energy or RED-S (see page 40); injury; burnout; and eventually, even full-blown eating disorders, such as anorexia and bulimia. These issues are incredibly common among distance runners—one study of women running NCAA Division I cross country and track found nearly half of them screened positive for the risk of eating disorders (Krebs et al. 2019). They've been brought to light in recent years by brave runners of all levels, including Mary Cain; Amelia Boone; and Molly Seidel, who says she'd never have won her bronze medal in the Olympic Marathon if she hadn't gone through treatment for her eating disorder (Kuzma 2021).

And I know the concerns aren't limited to college or pro athletes alone; they come up again and again among the runners I coach, and when I posted a video about body image on my YouTube channel, it got more views than any other by far. I know that some of this comes from a healthy place. After all, many people get into running as a way to lose weight and make positive lifestyle changes, but it's all too easy for that motivation to turn into one based on fear, obsession, and restriction.

I made significant shifts in my attitudes about this as my pro career progressed, but it came to a head again when I had Athens. The comparison game among pro athletes, sadly, doesn't end with a positive pregnancy test. While I ballooned all over and felt too sick to run, I stared sadly at the cute and well-formed baby bumps of other elites who were able to keep up their mileage until the day their water broke. When I saw people who lost their baby pounds pronto and were back to racing—and fast—months after giving birth, I dwelled on how different I looked and how far I was from them and from the runner I believed myself to be.

Thanks to all the runner mamas I've messaged, talked to, and coached, I now understand how common these feelings are. Everyone's journey is so different and as my example shows, can vary widely from one pregnancy to the next. You're low on sleep and high on hormones, so your emotions are primed to swell and surge. As a runner used to having so much control over your body, it's a strange sensation to essentially turn it over to another being, even one you want and love as much as your baby. When you take a step back, it's entirely understandable why you'd be struggling, and just knowing that can make it easier to extend grace to yourself.

As I've described in previous chapters, after a false start and another injury, I worked my way back into healthy postpartum running by changing my entire approach. I ditched the scale and focused on how I felt instead of how I looked, setting goals around nourishing myself instead of losing weight or cutting back. Of course, those old thoughts of restriction creep in from time to time—we're inundated with them, both from the running world and the larger culture. But now, I can recognize them for what they are and replace them with a healthy mindset. If you're having a hard time doing this, I hear you, and I want you to know that there's no shame in reaching out for support—be it from a dietitian, a sport psychologist, or a knowledgeable sports medicine physician. I've found them all extremely beneficial in the past. (And if you're in a crisis, you can always reach out to the National Eating Disorders Association Helpline at (800) 931-2237 or text "NEDA" to 741741.)

Forgive me for stepping up on my soapbox here, but I say it's time to do away once and for all with the idea of the "runner's body." What defines you as an athlete is all the stuff that's inside—the drive to set big goals, the courage to chase them down, and the thrill when you've succeeded. And while the time on the clock is one measure of progress, the most important metric is the progress you've made and the way you've grown as an athlete and a person along the way.

Remember, too, that when you're coming back from pregnancy, injury, disordered eating, or any other setback, your goal shouldn't be to reclaim who you were before. Rather, it's all about becoming your best self in the life and the body you're living in right now. Your goals and timelines may shift, and that's not giving up—it's embracing reality and rising up to meet it. With that as a foundation, you can move forward to achieve things you never believed possible.

Finding Her Power: Elise Cranny

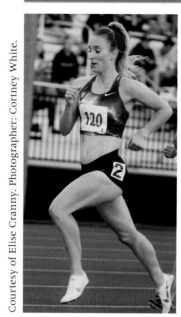

Courtesy of Elise Cranny. Photographer: Cortney White.

In 2020 and 2021—when many athletes were struggling to stay on track during the pandemic—Elise Cranny was dominating. The former Stanford middle-distance star improved her personal-best 5K time to 14:48:02 at a meet against only her teammates. She qualified for the Olympic Track & Field Trials in three events—the 1,500 meters, the 5,000 meters, and the 10,000 meters—then made the Olympic Track & Field Team in the 5,000 meters. In Tokyo, she made the final and finished 13th in a season-best 14:55:98.

The accomplishments were all the more rewarding because of the foundation they were built upon. Elise lost her period in high school, a fact her mother raised concerns about at the time. But it wasn't until her sophomore year at Stanford University, when she developed a sacral stress fracture, that Elise committed to giving up her restrictive eating habits and restoring it. "I thought, whoa, there are some serious underlying problems that are going to impact me for the rest of my life if I don't get this figured out," she says.

With her support team—including her family, dietitians, and psychologists—she began setting small process goals surrounding fueling. One day, it was adding a snack, and another, supplementing dinner with an extra half an avocado or sauce on her rice. Telling others about these goals and writing them down, separately from her training, helped her see progress and hold herself accountable.

The process wasn't always easy, nor was it linear. Even after her period came back, she still had several bone injuries as her body rebuilt from years of deficit. But she remained committed to healthy changes, and she urges other athletes to take the longer-term view. "Don't be discouraged," she says. "Have grace for your body."

Over time, as she regained strength, she put far less stock in what she saw in the mirror. Rather than tell her anything about her fitness, the shape and size of her body were leading her astray. "Appearance changes based on if you just ate a meal, how hydrated you are, where you are in your cycle—all of those things," she says. "This is a poor indicator of anything because my body looks completely different at different hours of the day."

Instead of a look, she began chasing a feeling—fit and empowered, like herself, but with a turbo boost. To remind herself, she puts positive mantras on repeat: "You're feeling strong, you're racing strong, and that's what's most important," she says. "I no longer felt like I was holding things together, on the brink of getting injured."

Once she got her period back, reading *ROAR* and tracking her cycle helped Elise better maximize her physiology. "The more we understand it, the more we can use it to our advantage," she says. She knows she'll feel bloated and have trouble sleeping right before getting her period. Some workouts at that time feel harder; she views them as opportunities to practice for tough races. On the flip side, when a competition happens to fall soon after getting her period, she thrives on the added confidence that brings.

When she's tempted to slip into comparisons on social media or at the starting line, Elise reminds herself that no single body type leads to running success. "That was actually really freeing for me; why am I trying to do what someone else is doing?" she says. Even if she followed the exact same training and fueling strategy as one of her teammates or competitors, they probably wouldn't look the same anyway.

This attitude has not only improved her performance, but it's also restored her love of the sport. "This is the body I've been given. How can I focus on my own journey and do the best I can with it?" she says. "This is a fun process of learning more about myself, tapping into my potential, seeing how I can be at my best, and enjoying it along the way."

FROM BARRIER TO BREAKTHROUGH

Thanks to the hard work of researchers such as Dr. Stacy Sims, we know more about women's bodies—and their athletic greatness—than ever. Here are some ideas for harnessing your physiology.

Barrier

I've never thought about how my hormones or my cycle affects my running, but now I'm curious to learn more.

Breakthrough Goals

Choose one or more.

I will do the following:

- Begin tracking my period and comparing it to my running log to see whether there are any correlations between where I'm at in my cycle and how I feel
- Read Dr. Sims' books and follow her on social media (She's on Instagram at @drstacysims and @womenarenotsmallmen.)
- Ask my health care provider how my birth control method affects my cycle if applicable

---

Barrier

The symptoms that go along with my cycle are so bad that they derail my running.

Breakthrough Goals

Choose one or more.

I will do the following:

- Begin tracking my period so I know the timing of my cycle and can better prepare for the down days
- Consider planning my training around my cycle, taking extra rest or easy running days at the time when I feel the worst
- Increase my focus on hydration with both water and electrolytes shortly before my period
- Experiment with seed cycling or Dr. Sims' PMS protocol on page 63
- Talk with my health care provider about ways to minimize my symptoms

Barrier

I'm nervous about getting my period on race day.

Breakthrough Goals

Choose one or more.

I will do the following:

- Track my period so I can start to see the effects of my cycle and predict when my period will come
- Remember that many athletes race better on their periods
- Practice with several types of period products to see what works best
- Have an entire plan for handling my period on race day, including the products I'll use and when and how I'll change them (See page 65 for more about how to do this.)

Barrier

I don't have confidence I can achieve my goals because I don't "look like" a runner.

Breakthrough Goals

Choose one or more.

I will do the following:

- Reread Elise Cranny's and Neely's stories and remind myself that successful runners come in all shapes and sizes
- Write down the feeling I'm aiming for—strong, powerful, and ready to run well—and remind myself that's the goal, not a certain weight or physique
- Do a social media audit (If I follow runners or fitness accounts on these platforms, I'll make sure they don't all look the same.)
- Experiment with not weighing myself or looking in the mirror at the body parts that bother me
- Reach out to a dietitian, nutritionist, or sport psychology expert for support

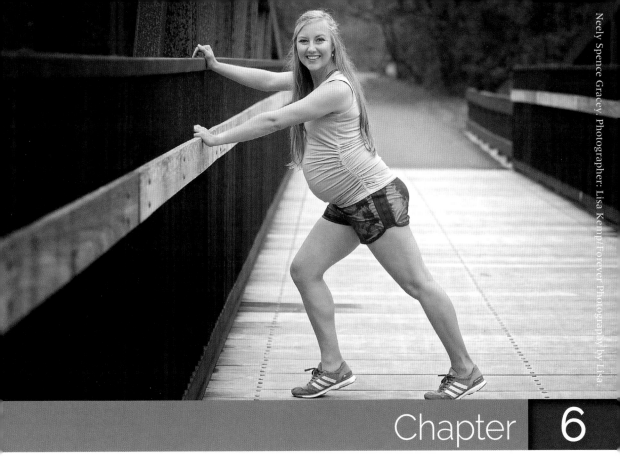

Chapter | 6

Ready, Set, Grow

" Even if I knew for certain that I would be a better or faster runner if my life had looked differently, I wouldn't change anything. Would running have been easier for me if I hadn't had kids? Almost certainly. Would my life be half as fulfilling? Definitely no. And though I don't believe in 'balance,' I definitely do support well-rounded lifestyles. Because while it's hard, there's nothing better. "

Sara Vaughn, pro runner, realtor, and mom of four

When I put my pro running career on pause to have my first child in 2017, I was excited—but terrified. I looked up to other elite mama runners, such as Kara Goucher and Alysia Montaño, who were gracious enough to answer my (many) questions. However, I still found precious little information about how to navigate this new and challenging period.

Fortunately, things are changing. More doctors and exercise scientists are studying active moms and moms-to-be, providing evidence-based guidance for running during and after pregnancy. More elite athletes than ever have returned to the sport at the highest levels as moms, their performances refuting outdated thinking. And social media, provided we use it productively, gives us all the chance to connect and share experiences and advice.

Since those early, anxious days, I've made it my mission to educate myself about these topics, then share what I know with the athletes I coach and the public. (At the time I'm writing this, my assistant coaches and I are working with 12 pregnant athletes!) Of course, I hope to provide useful information to guide women through. But more than anything, I want other runner moms to know you're not alone, that you're understood and supported.

GREAT EXPECTATIONS

From the time Dillon and I decided to start a family, I had a clear vision for how my first pregnancy would go. I'd run right up until my delivery date—after all, I'm a pro, and that's what my mom and sisters had done. Afterward, I'd start slowly at the six-week mark but swiftly gain steam. I'd be back to top competitive form quickly, as pros such as Kara Goucher and Gwen Jorgensen had before me.

Reality set in right after I stared in shock at those two lines on the pregnancy test. Beginning at eight weeks, I felt nauseated and strongly averse to food, except for pizza, watermelon, and ice cream. My back ached, so I stopped running completely after 18 weeks, and round ligament pain kept me from strength training. Summer's heat, the deviation from my typical diet, and swirling hormones left me low on energy and motivation to do much cross-training. I had a supportive partner and medical team, including an obstetrician who was a runner and understood my challenges. Still, I couldn't help but beat myself up about my sedentary habits and weight gain.

Athens arrived healthy and strong, but as I've already touched on, my postpartum route back was far more winding and difficult than I expected. It took a year and a half before I even began to find my footing and make my way back to a starting line, let alone a triumphant finish.

After the Houston Marathon and the Olympic Marathon Trials in the summer of 2020, I began to feel like the athlete I had been—and in fact, an even stronger one. But like so much else that year, things didn't unfold as expected. I've already explained how my second pregnancy wasn't exactly planned. The ease with which it happened, by the way, is something I don't take for granted; I know many people face immense struggles in their quest to become parents, and my heart goes out to them.

This experience was dramatically different. I ate normally, with the exception of a few extra chocolate chip cookies. I was able to keep running, and I even did Fartlek workouts and longer runs through 14 weeks. I can't say which was the cause and which the effect, but I had far less stress and more faith in my body and myself.

Time will tell how my full recovery will pan out. My athletic timeline will look different than I'd thought. But know this—I fully intend to continue chasing down my goals. Originally, I'd planned to compete through 2024, then complete my family. Now, I see no ceiling on how long I can keep aiming for my best.

Since I first announced my pregnancy with Athens, I've communicated with hundreds if not thousands of other current and soon-to-be runner moms. The connection between us is intense as we make our way through this surprisingly uncharted territory. The information in this chapter will, I hope, make those conversations accessible to more people, offering practical guidance to those who feel as overwhelmed and alone as I once did. Every pregnancy is different, but I hope there is at least one helpful takeaway for you from this chapter.

Most importantly, though, I want you to recognize that this phase doesn't represent the end or even a step away from your career as an athlete. Rather, it places you firmly in the center of an even bigger, more beautiful running story. From sports bras to running marathons to Title IX, women have made and continue to make breakthroughs in sport. Motherhood is the next great frontier.

For a long time, women worked and then became mothers. Athletes competed, then retired to start a family. Increasingly, though, we're pushing back and setting our own timelines. Rather than choosing to give up one goal for another, we're merely hitting pause, reserving the right to resume when we're ready.

Yes, it's tough to "do it all," but what if we don't have to? What if partners step up and parent fifty-fifty? What if we had more affordable and accessible childcare? What if we had parental leave allowing for bonding and healing without loss of income?

We are just at the beginning of a breakthrough in these areas. While activists and organizations work toward policy changes, we can all be a part of this movement. If we don't hold ourselves back, we show ourselves—and everyone else, including our children—what's possible.

Nothing worthwhile is easy. Success always takes time. If you're pregnant or a new mom, you may not hit the performances you want this year. It might take two or three or even four years—or longer—to reach your goals. But I'm here to tell you that you're incredible and you can accomplish great things, both as a mom and an athlete. You deserve to enjoy the process, take pride in your efforts, and rebuild in the time that feels right and not forced. Even—and perhaps even more so—as a mom, pursuing your potential can change your life.

STOP, SLOW, OR GO?

The number one question I get is, can I continue running while I'm pregnant? The unsatisfying answer is, it depends. My strongest advice is to work with your doctor and listen to your body, practicing flexibility and grace.

First, a few basic facts. There's a growing consensus among medical experts that exercise is extremely beneficial for pregnant women and their babies. "Women who can exercise during pregnancy tend to have healthier pregnancies, lower risk of high blood pressure, lower risk of gestational diabetes, better labors, and better postpartum recoveries," says Dr. Christine H. Abair, a runner and board-certified obstetrician who practices at Boulder Medical Center. (She's my supportive obstetrician whom I mentioned earlier.) The American College of Obstetricians and Gynecologists agrees and released guidelines in April 2020 recommending that doctors encourage their pregnant patients to start or continue a fitness routine (ACOG Committee on Obstetric Practice 2020).

Of course, running is a high-impact, demanding sport. Most women who were runners before becoming pregnant can safely continue to train about the same number of days per week (Kuhrt et al. 2018), albeit at a less aggressive pace and distance, Dr. Abair says. But your doctor might recommend you switch to cross-training or even rest altogether during pregnancy for a few reasons, including a high risk for preterm labor or bleeding, placenta previa, or a short cervix.

If your doctor says you and your baby are healthy but still discourages running, I recommend seeking a second opinion, preferably from a doctor who's familiar with athletes. I recognize this might be easier in some places than others. I have had athletes reach out from cultures where women's running isn't yet accepted and who have more barriers to overcome. On the flip side, in other societies, active moms are better supported by both society and policies, such as family leave. My hope is that by openly discussing these topics, we can move the needle in a positive direction everywhere.

The other basic fact is that for this brief period, the most important job your body has is growing a baby. You might have complications leading your doctor to limit your activity, or you could just feel too nauseated, fatigued, or uncomfortable to run. While we're conditioned to push through pain as athletes, there are also times when it pays to hold back, and pregnancy is certainly one of them. Some discomfort is normal, of course, but running through pelvic or back pain may extend your timeline for getting back to running afterward, according to Dr. Sara Tanza, a pelvic floor physical therapist at Pelvic Potential in Santa Cruz, California, who's worked with several pro runners.

During my pregnancy with Athens, I wondered whether I was too mentally weak to run or I just didn't care enough—had I lost my competitive edge forever? Looking back now, this is what I'd tell myself and now I'll tell you: *All this is temporary. You are a great mom. You and your doctors together will focus on your top priorities, which are your baby's health and your own. If your body needs all its energy to grow an entirely complete and perfect little human, that is absolutely enough.*

BABY ON BOARD

As athletes, we're highly attuned to the way our bodies change and adapt as we train. The same miraculous, flexible set of organs and systems also shift to promote your baby's development. Some changes definitely influence the way your body responds to running and other exercises, including the following:

- As your belly grows larger, your center of gravity shifts, which challenges your balance, especially later in your pregnancy. I always avoided rocky and icy terrain, staying on the treadmill if the weather was bad. Plus, you'll have to modify your strength moves—I personally couldn't squat with weight or do hinging exercises, such as Romanian deadlifts.
- Your changing spinal curve increases the forces across your back and joints.
- Hormonal shifts loosen your hips and pelvis to let baby grow and eventually, to pass through.
- Your blood volume increases, and so does the amount your heart pumps with each stroke.
- Your heart rate rises, too, meaning the amount of blood that pumps through your body every minute significantly increases. In fact, your resting heart rate may be as much as 20 to 25 percent higher than your baseline by the time you give birth.
- You might take more frequent, shallow breaths as your baby simultaneously presses on your diaphragm and adds to your need for oxygen (ACOG Committee on Obstetric Practice 2018; Meah, Davies, and Davenport 2020).
- Hormones, such as progesterone and human chorionic gonadotropin, which rise in early pregnancy, produce an urge to pee. And as your baby grows, so might pressure on your bladder or bowels, further increasing that gotta-go feeling—especially when you add the pounding of running.

TRAINING AND TRYING

What if you're not pregnant yet but want to be? I've coached many athletes who were trying to conceive but were also signed up for a goal race.

Dr. Abair says there's nothing wrong with that plan: "As long as there are no pre-existing conditions that would make you high risk, you are not doing fertility treatments, and you're consistently getting your period, then it's a green light to keeping going with both volume and intensity in training," she says. While your doctor can answer any questions you have about your specific situation, it helps to know there's no evidence that training increases your risk of miscarriage (Davenport et al. 2019).

Because it often takes time—an average of 6 to 12 months—to get pregnant, you might even make it through one or two training cycles while you're working on it. If you're used to running regularly, continuing to pursue your other goals can give you a sense of control during a time that's often stressful, Dr. Abair points out. And the same healthy lifestyle, with adequate fueling and rest, can increase your odds of success in both pursuits.

One caveat I'll add is that it's extra important in this situation to keep things in perspective and not let your running become a source of stress. Instead, view it as a win-win. No matter how the timing works out, you're dedicating yourself to two big, important goals—and that, in itself, is awesome.

So it's no wonder running might feel different—and more difficult—while you're expecting. Some days, you'll feel great, and some days, you'll struggle. There are so many factors that contribute, such as where baby's positioned. (I often developed side stitches, likely because Rome was right under my ribs.) Sometimes, there's no reason other than your body diverting its resources into growing a human.

RUNNING FOR TWO

While running went far better for me the second time around, fatigue is still real and present. I can run 100-plus-mile weeks and not feel nearly as drained as I do when pregnant. And then there's morning sickness, which for some people (like me!) becomes an all-day affair.

Those complications, along with the physical changes previously outlined, definitely make running while pregnant challenging at times. But there's a lot you can do to boost your energy levels, fuel your motivation, and just plain feel better.

- *Embrace a slower pace.* Even if you still do some faster running, your overall pace will likely creep downward. During pregnancy, my easy runs averaged anywhere from 30 seconds to a full two and a half minutes per mile slower than the rest of the time.

- *Follow your breath.* You can use heart rate to gauge your intensity—per ACOG, it's best to stay under 80 percent of your maximum. If you've heard that old advice about keeping it under 140 beats per minute, you should know that guideline was based on little evidence and has since been thoroughly debunked, but somehow, some doctors are still stuck on it (Mottola et al. 2018)! Even with the newer guidelines, however, some people still don't know what their max heart rate is. And because your heart rate is affected by pregnancy anyway, I find it easier to use rating of perceived exertion (RPE) and keep my efforts at a maximum of 8 out of 10. As long as your breath stays controlled, both you and the baby are getting enough oxygen.

- *Play with speed.* Again, with your doctor's OK to run, you can keep doing workouts as you feel able—with my second pregnancy, I did them through 14 weeks. Rather than structured track intervals or tempo runs at a set pace, try Fartleks and run for time. I like doing a combination of 30-, 60-, and 90-second intervals, then jogging as long as needed in between to fully recover.

- *Break it up.* Many days, especially later in pregnancy, an easy jog is plenty challenging. Add walk or rest breaks into your runs if your heart rate increases or your breathing becomes labored, Dr. Abair says.

- *Keep a routine.* Aim to head out around the same time each day, at an hour when you typically feel better. This might be in the afternoon if you have morning sickness or early in the day if fatigue is your primary issue.

- *Drink plenty of fluids.* Hydration is critically important for pregnant women (Healthline n.d.). Getting plenty of water and electrolyte-enhanced beverages keeps all your body's functions running smoothly and prevents you from overheating, which can be risky for you and your baby.

- *Power up.* Always eat before and after running, and make sure your meal or snack includes a quick-digesting carbohydrate source. For longer runs, I'd make sure to tote energy chews or an electrolyte drink with calories. And I'd snack again afterward. In fact, running always went better for me when I snacked throughout the day, avoiding being too hungry or full. I'd carry cheese, crackers, and grapes or apple slices and peanut butter around in a plastic container and nibble as I could.

- *Stay cool.* Avoid extreme heat; try to run during cooler parts of the day or on a treadmill if that's the best way to escape hot, humid conditions.

- *But not too cold.* Keeping warm in subzero temperatures can add excess stress to your body. When the temperature drops, hit the treadmill, or try the warmer parts of the day if your schedule's flexible. Also, if you live where it's snowy and icy, stick to roads and paths that are plowed and salted to reduce your risk of falling. Don't be afraid to run inside or cross-train instead if you feel at all unsafe.

- *Snooze away.* Get plenty of sleep at night, and when possible, squeeze a nap into your schedule. That few minutes of extra shut-eye can boost your energy and improve your recovery.

- *Keep it smooth.* In addition to avoiding ice and snow, you'll likely want to steer clear of routes that are rocky, uneven, or otherwise treacherous. Between your shifting balance and, later, inability to see your feet, the risk of falling is just too great.

These techniques can help, but if you're still dragging, it can be tough to know when rest is best and when powering through will make you feel better in the long run. My rule of thumb is to stick to your exercise plan as often as possible but if you start and still feel drained after 10 minutes, turn back or walk home. Sometimes, you might surprise yourself and decide to continue; other days, it's best to heed your body's warnings and call it early.

Know, too, that if you're super drained at first, you may actually feel a surge of energy in the second trimester. That's also when your morning sickness may lift (I say may because with Athens, mine didn't, but for many people, it does improve). Of course, this occurs as you're also noticing more of the other physical changes associated with pregnancy. Many people hit a "sweet spot" around 12 to 20 weeks when they can enjoy feeling pregnant and run a little more freely.

Regardless, though, extend yourself plenty of grace. There's so much going on that you can't control, and even the things within your power might not work for you in the same way they usually do. During pregnancy, I found I could do everything "right" and still have a terrible run or be totally off my game but feel great once I got started. It's a good time to practice going with the flow and doing the best with what you have on any given day, knowing that sometimes, the best thing you can do is rest.

A RUNNER'S REGISTRY

With my first pregnancy, I didn't bother buying maternity running clothes. I would definitely advise picking up a few basics as well as some sized-up running clothes for during and after pregnancy so you're not squeezing into your previous size and feeling uncomfortable and upset (or stretching out your favorite crop tights).

YOUR NEW RUNNING PARTNER

Taking your kiddo along for the run is one of the best ways for women to model a healthy lifestyle, says Christie Foster, a Colorado Springs–based pediatric physician's assistant. Plus, it helps busy moms reach their goals too.

Of course, the first question is, when is it safe to start bringing your little one along—and how do you start? Choosing the right stroller is only one part of the equation. There's a lot more you can do to make the experience of running together safe and comfortable for you and your child.

Timing is key: "Walking with—and keeping—your baby in a stroller with a car-seat adaptor or in a stroller that has a reclined position is a great way to get active those first few months after giving birth," Foster says. "However, it is important to wait until your baby is around six months of age to run with the stroller."

By then, most babies are sitting with little or no support and have enough core and neck control to withstand bumps, jostles, and turns. Sleeping in a semi-upright position is never safe for a young baby because of the risk of sudden infant death syndrome, or SIDS—but that risk declines at six months. They're also fans of movement and likely to enjoy the ride, she says.

Though that's a general guideline, Foster recommends talking with your pediatrician first; some babies might be ready earlier, whereas some may need to wait until closer to eight months.

Once you're given the go-ahead, dress your baby for the weather. That includes a good slather with sunscreen—don't forget to apply it to little feet that might stick out of the stroller. If the forecast calls for wind or rain, bring a shield. Use the safety brake anytime you stop, and consider a safety strap for your wrist, especially at first.

Here's a few more tips from my experience. I always made sure I took care of everyone's needs before heading out for a stroller run. Athens was fed and burped and had a clean diaper—that way, he was more comfortable, and so was I.

Between getting ready and stopping along the way, know that stroller runs will always take longer than you think; if you have 45 minutes in your schedule, you'll likely be able to get in only a 30-minute jog. That's all right because it's generally best to stay closer to home, especially until you're a bit more confident.

I also packed a special toy or, when he was older, played games with him on the run. And if all else failed, I'd give him my phone. Athens actually didn't like stroller running at first—he'd cry almost every time—but by the time he was about one and a half, he couldn't wait to go out with me.

"Remember to be flexible with both your baby and yourself, and enjoy the freedom of being able to run on your own schedule with your new favorite training partner," Foster says.

So in addition to the baby clothes and nursery decor, consider putting a few products in the cart just for you.

- My favorite maternity running gear so far has come from Cadenshae (which has also worked with Alysia Montaño's &Mother nonprofit organization to support mama athletes), H&M maternity activewear, PinkBlush maternity activewear, and Target.

- The Maternity FITsplint, developed and sold by runner and certified medical exercise specialist Celeste Goodson at ReCORE Fitness, provides core and pelvic support and reduces strain on your back while running. She also sells a postnatal version for supporting your core muscles after you give birth.

- Your feet often grow and swell during pregnancy, so you might need to buy a slightly larger pair of running shoes. I also found that postpartum, I needed more cushioning than I did before to avoid aches, pains, and injuries.

- Colorado-based, woman-owned Motherlove makes a great belly salve for pregnant women's growing bodies and a nipple cream to ease soreness and cracking while breastfeeding.

- A stroller. First of all, don't feel like you *must* own a running stroller if you don't want one—it's OK to keep your sport something that's just for you! Personally, I like to train mostly on my own, but I do have a running stroller for the occasional family jog. My go-to is the Thule Urban Glide 2—it's more aerodynamic and compact than other models I've tried and has a lower handle that's perfect for my height (five feet, four inches). When you're shopping around, consider size, smoothness, and whether the stroller has a car-seat attachment.

THE LONG ROAD

If I thought I felt alone and uncertain during pregnancy, returning to running after Athens was born presented an even greater challenge. While Dr. Abair continued to be incredibly supportive, our infrequent postpartum visits weren't enough to address what came next for me.

In many ways, postnatal running is like returning from an injury—and depending on what your birth experience was like, a relatively serious one involving surgery or torn muscles in your pelvic floor. In other aspects, however, it's entirely different. When you're injured, your body is still your own. But after pregnancy, you're essentially an entirely different human—one who's now responsible for tending to a small being. And you're doing all this on minimal sleep, which we all know is essential to recovery.

When I came back after Athens, I thought I did everything "right." I took three weeks off entirely, then began light biking and elliptical alongside a core-training routine with Goodson of ReCORE Fitness. When I was cleared by Dr. Abair and Goodson to run, I started with a 10 by one-minute walk, one-minute run. By the time Athens was six months old, I worked my way back to 70-mile weeks while breastfeeding, making sure I was eating and hydrating well so my milk supply wasn't affected.

But when I weaned him at nine months, my hormonal shifts set me back. My first postpartum period lasted two weeks and felt like the flu. I developed shin splints, something I hadn't had since my early days in the sport. Reduced levels of the hormone relaxin tightened my left hip, then caused me to compensate in a way I believe led to the stress fracture on the opposite side.

This was the low point for me—the one I mentioned way back at the beginning of the book—when I was doubting myself and my path, wondering whether I'd ever return to the pro ranks. At my one-year checkup, I was in tears as I despondently listed my frustrations. Dr. Abair was so empathetic and emphasized that sometimes, it takes up to four years to fully rebuild on a cellular level from pregnancy. Suddenly, instead of feeling behind, I was reassured. I was only one-fourth of the way through a four-year process. There was so much more improvement ahead if I could stay patient and diligent.

A year later, I was in a completely different spot, mentally and physically. I was able to fulfill my goals of qualifying for and lining up at the Olympic Marathon Trials. That summer, thanks to the healthy mindset and fueling as I described in chapter 4, I was on track to exceed my previous performances when I found out I was pregnant again. While the arrival of little Rome was another adjustment to my plans, I now knew I had what it took to rebuild yet again.

POSTPARTUM PROGRESS

As more and more moms set their sights on athletic goals, experts such as Goodson have stepped in to fill the gap between postpartum care and regular training. Through

COMMON COMPLICATIONS

In a perfect world, all new moms would have access to a team of professionals looking out for their and their baby's health—not just an obstetrician but a certified medical exercise specialist, such as Goodson; a running coach trained in prenatal and postnatal training; and a pelvic floor physical therapist, such as Dr. Tanza, who is a health care provider who can assess and examine you inside and out to prevent and treat issues with these very important muscles.

While not everyone has the time and resources to pursue these services before problems develop, it's important to know what's normal and when you should push for more medical treatment. Some common complications that can delay your return to normal activities include the following:

- Diastasis recti, or excessive stretching of the tissue (linea alba) between the rectus abdominis muscles
- Tears in your pelvic floor muscles
- Pelvic organ prolapse, a condition caused by weak or damaged pelvic floor muscles that allow organs, such as your uterus and bladder, to drop down into or out of your vagina

Watch for these warning signs of pelvic floor dysfunction, and talk to a pelvic floor physical therapist or doctor if you develop them:

- Leaking urine or stool when you're resting, coughing, sneezing, walking, running, or jumping
- Pain with sex
- A bulge between your abdominal muscles when you sit up
- Sensations of heaviness in your vagina or rectum, as if tampons are falling out
- Pain in your pelvis or abdomen

While these issues are common, they're not normal, meaning that you don't have to simply cope with them. Treatment can not only improve your health and well-being now, but it can also ward off running injuries later on because these muscles act as incredibly important stabilizers, Dr. Tanza says.

her pre- and postnatal fitness program, she's helped everyone from pro athletes to new runners enjoy the sport after giving birth.

Healing times vary greatly, she notes, depending on your hormones, genetics, how difficult a birth you had, any complications you develop, and how much sleep you're able to get. While many women are cleared to run again at 6 weeks, the latest international guidelines actually suggest waiting up to 12 weeks provided you don't have the red-flag symptoms listed previously (Goom, Donnelly, and Brockwell 2019).

Of course, guidelines are generalities, and working with your doctor or another health care provider is key. If you can see a specialist, such as a pelvic floor physical therapist, that's generally best; your doctor may tell you, for instance, that your C-section incision is healed and then sends you on your way, but there's a lot more that goes into rebuilding the underlying muscles.

Dr. Tanza often clears runners to introduce drills and light jumping at 8 weeks and running at 12 weeks if they're healthy enough. Some people are cleared to start sooner or need to wait longer based on injuries sustained to the pelvic floor during vaginal birth or the abdominal muscles during C-section, ongoing pelvic pain, pelvic floor heaviness, or continued incontinence.

And regardless, that doesn't mean resting completely for months, then going out to run five miles. Rebuilding your body requires a stepwise progression. Here's the best advice I've received and offered about this path.

Start With Strength

Pregnancy stretches and weakens all your core muscles, from your pelvic floor to your abs and back, and both C-sections and vaginal births can cause additional damage. A program such as Goodson's ReCORE (available online if you can't train one-on-one with someone like her) is designed for just this purpose. It starts with basic deep breathing to reengage stretched-out, weak core muscles. From there, you'll progress to working surrounding, stabilizing muscles in the upper and lower body. Then you'll add weights and reintroduce your body gently to impact to not further damage healing tissues and to give the pelvic floor a chance to adapt.

Walk

At the same time you're rebuilding your core, you can start with low-impact activities, such as walking. After I had Athens, the first thing we did when we got home was a slow, short walk around the block. I did this almost every day, gradually increasing until I could walk four miles. Dr. Tanza advises her athletes to build up their walk to about double the amount of time they'd typically run, which would mean, for example, walking for an hour and a half if most of your weekday runs were about 45 minutes. And I'd do all this while wearing the Post-Natal FITsplint from Goodson; she recommends keeping it on up to eight hours a day for at least four to six weeks, above your scar if you had a C-section (though you'll want to check with your doctor first).

Add Hill Repeats

Some women can go straight from walking to run-walking. But there's no harm in taking it slower, and if you have any of the red-flag symptoms previously listed, your health care providers might wait to clear you to resume pounding your feet into the ground. Goodson advises moving on to walking hill repeats, which add aerobic intensity while building leg and hip strength, all with less impact than running. The stair stepper and elliptical work well at this phase too.

Sprinkle in Run Intervals

Once you've made it to this point—and remember, there's no rush—you can flip to chapter 15 for a run-walk training plan. Begin this when you've been cleared to run.

Concentrate on Cadence

After time off from running, hormonal shifts, and differences in your body composition, your risk of injury may be somewhat higher. One way to reduce this risk is to focus on cadence. Most GPS watches have this data marker to help guide you; I recommend aiming for around 180 strides per minute, though if you're far below that, bring it up 5

EATING FOR YOU

If you read chapter 4 on nutrition, you know the importance of proper fueling for running. All this takes on added importance during pregnancy and postpartum and while breastfeeding. Yes, you may be running less, but you're also growing and nourishing a human.

Many new moms are eager to drop their pregnancy pounds, but cutting calories places you at high risk of RED-S—relative energy deficiency in sport—which we discuss at length on page 40. Particularly at this vulnerable time, insufficient energy can delay your healing, harm your bones, and affect your future fertility. And it can also interfere with your baby's growth and development (Goom, Donnelly, and Brockwell 2019).

Your doctor or a registered dietitian can provide personalized advice on your eating plan. Generally, rather than thinking about restriction, I recommend an overall strategy of whole, healthy foods to provide the nutrients you and your baby need to thrive. If you're looking for things to focus on, I suggest the following:

- *Prioritizing protein.* In addition to promoting recovery from your training, protein and the amino acids that make it up are essential for your baby's development. Aim for at least 75 to 100 grams per day, although you might also need more depending on your weight and how much you're running.

- *Finding folate.* This B vitamin is critical to your baby's development, and many people don't get enough. Look for a prenatal vitamin containing folate, not folic acid; it's easier to absorb. And eat plenty of folate-rich foods, such as lentils, avocado, spinach, and cooked asparagus.

- *Seeking supplemental help.* About that prenatal vitamin, ask your doctor for more details about the best one for you and also discuss other common deficiencies. Runners' needs for iron, essential fatty acids, vitamin D, and magnesium are often different than those of sedentary people, so check whether you should get blood tests or shore up your stores.

- *Adding electrolytes.* Not only do these essential minerals keep your muscles firing properly, but they're also critical for bone health because they help our bodies better absorb and maintain calcium levels. And both pregnancy and breastfeeding increase the amount of calcium you need! So swapping out every other bottle of water for an electrolyte-enhanced drink can protect your skeleton during this critical period (Hew-Butler, Stuempfle, and Hoffman 2013; Salari and Abdollahi 2014).

percent or so at a time. This boosts your efficiency, prevents overstriding, and reduces your ground contact time, all of which protect your bones, tendons, and joints. Plus, it gives you a metric to focus on that isn't pace or distance.

Note: Postpartum running is rarely a straightforward, linear progression. It's important to listen to your body and spend as much time as you need focusing on each phase. Don't be afraid to repeat or step back your exercises or redo a week of run-walk progressions if that's what feels manageable to you at the time. Any potential boost to your fitness is far outweighed by the risk of getting injured by doing too much, too soon.

Your time and energy are divided right now, and that's perfectly fine—you won't get those early baby days back, so soak them up, knowing your competitive goals will always be there for you later. I wrote the following in a letter to my future self six days after I found out about my second pregnancy: *Do not rush things. Go at your own pace. Listen to your body and your heart. Forcing things gets you nowhere, but being patient and slowing down take you so far when the time is right.*

MORE MAMA MATTERS

As your body shifts from a pregnancy and birth focus into mom mode, there are a few other notable changes that may affect your running.

- Your size and shape may be in flux for a while. It's a good idea to have a few pieces of running gear that are in between—larger than you wore before but smaller than your maternity clothes (by this time, you're sick of those anyway). Thankfully, high-waisted clothing is in style, which helps keep everything a lot more comfortable!

- As the higher blood volume you had during pregnancy decreases, excess fluid has to go somewhere. Frequently, it comes out as sweat. Know that you might soak through a few more running tanks and shorts, even before you start your workout, and that you probably can't get away with a quick rinse or a dry shampoo afterward to clean up. This is another reason it's very important to stay hydrated. I take a water bottle to bed, and when I'm feeding the baby, I make sure I'm drinking too.

- Speaking of fluids, you'll probably find yourself leaking blood and urine for a while after birth. The same types of products you use for your period, including pads and period clothing, will serve you well here too. (Doctors typically recommend waiting at least six weeks before using tampons; check with your doctor first to stay on the safe side.) With Rome, I waited to start anything more than easy walking and light core work until I stopped bleeding regularly. Until then, I realized my body was still doing a lot of healing.

- If you gave birth by C-section, keep tabs on your scar. Depending on the type of incision and how it heals, the surrounding muscles, organs, and other systems can be affected (Goom, Donnelly, and Brockwell 2019). Scar mobilization can help—something physical therapists, chiropractors, or other specialists can guide you on.

ALL ABOUT BREASTFEEDING

Most health organizations—including the American College of Obstetricians and Gynecologists (ACOG Committee on Obstetric Practice 2018) and the American Academy of Pediatrics (Johnston et al. 2012)—recommend breastfeeding exclusively for six months and alongside other foods for a year or longer. Of course, many families make a different choice for various reasons. You have to do what's best for you and your baby, but know that you can absolutely make breastfeeding work with your running.

After I had Athens, I was able to sustain up to 70-mile weeks and had an adequate milk supply. And I'm not alone. When Olympic marathoner Aliphine Tuliamuk reached out on Instagram in June 2021 to ask about others' experiences, elite mama runners from all over weighed in. Alysia Montaño, for instance, noted that she had won two national titles and even broke an American record in the 800 meters while breastfeeding.

Research on this topic is limited, but one study of runners found 84 percent of those who ran competitively before pregnancy continued while breastfeeding and most felt running had no detrimental effects (Bø et al. 2017). To make breastfeeding and training more effective and comfortable do the following:

- *Fuel properly.* As I keep coming back to, you need even more energy than normal if you're training and feeding both yourself and another human. The average woman needs an additional 400 to 500 calories while breastfeeding, and remember, as a runner, you're not average. Check with your doctor or a dietitian if you have specific questions about how much you need, but rest assured it's more than if you were doing either of these things in isolation.

- *Hydrate, then hydrate some more.* I always drank plenty of water before running and throughout the day, and if I were running for an hour or more, I'd take water with me. Even after a 16-mile-long run in fairly hot conditions, I never had any problem feeding Athens as soon as I got home.

- *Stay consistent.* Milk production is a supply-and-demand issue—in addition to ensuring your body has the raw materials to produce it, you have to continue signaling to your system that it's required. I would always try to feed Athens or pump at least once every four hours. If he wasn't up and ready to eat before a long run, for instance, I would pump. Not only was it a lot more comfortable to start my run with less-full breasts, but it also ensured that I would continue making milk on schedule. With Rome, I upgraded my pump to one that allowed me to use only one side—this helped me balance out times when he fell asleep after nursing on one breast. It's also battery operated, so it's easier to take on the go!

- *Switch up your sports bra.* You might find that a bra that's more supportive than compressive—and in a size that fits you now, not before pregnancy—goes a long way in making you feel better on the run. There are even nursing sports bras, from Cadenshae and others, that offer appropriate support and easy access. I also add disposable breastfeeding pads to soak up any milk that may dribble out on the run.

I've had plenty of athletes run personal bests while breastfeeding. In fact, weaning is often what takes a little more time to adjust to because your hormone levels shift again before restabilizing. Sometimes, your life situation—or your child's preferences—lead you to stop breastfeeding earlier than planned, and it's always something you can adjust to and work through. But if you have a choice in the matter, I recommend trying to time weaning between races, during the natural break in your training cycle.

MAMA MINDSET

The significant hormonal shifts you're going through during pregnancy and soon afterward absolutely influence your mood. All the while, you're balancing lots of change and uncertainty. Although building a family is a happy time, transformation can be uncomfortable, and you're likely concerned about how you'll parent or what a second (or third or fourth) child means for your household.

Just like in any long race or training block, you might hit points when you're feeling lower than others. Fortunately, as an athlete, you can draw on your experience tolerating discomfort and overcoming obstacles. To stay positive both around the time of pregnancy and as you continue balancing your running with your family life, you can do the following.

Adjust Your Goals

For me, hitting pause on my pro career—knowing I would return to my running goals soon—was useful. "I think the best mindset is to focus on being healthy," Dr. Abair says. "Pregnancy is not a time when you are going to hit your PR, but it is a great time to just get out there and keep moving."

Set Small Milestones

Give yourself mini goals en route to your bigger dreams. Celebrate the end of the first trimester. Applaud yourself for reaching the 20-week scan and halfway point. The 24-week mark—when your baby is viable—is a huge milestone! The third trimester begins, and the finish line is in sight. Marking these occasions can keep you present, in the moment, and grateful.

Make a Mantra

We'll talk more about these motivating phrases in chapter 9, but in brief, you can repeat them aloud or in writing to lift your spirits. Some that work well for pregnancy are "I am here for my baby," "This work is important," and "Eyes on the prize."

Find Role Models

Social media can be a wonderful place to share stories and tips, but it can also turn into a giant comparison trap, presenting highlight reels that leave you questioning yourself and your progression. My advice is to mute or unfollow any accounts that make you feel bad (you can always return to them later). Besides having personal conversations with other runner moms, I found it most useful to follow those who were a few years ahead in the process. Amazing athletes such as Sara Vaughn; Alysia Montaño; and Stephanie Bruce, who ran her personal-best marathon when her younger son was four years old, showed me they didn't put limits on themselves—and neither should I.

Seek Support

No mom can do it all, and she especially can't go it alone. Be your own advocate in this regard, planning ahead as well as asking for what you need when it arises. People want to help and like it when you're specific with your requests! I found myself much better at this with Rome than with Athens. Dillon took some time off, and my in-laws visited. And I was clear about what would be most helpful; for instance, I often wanted to do small tasks, such as clean out the dishwasher myself, but instead asked them to watch both kids for a few minutes afterward so I could take a shower. Outsource what you can—get friends to bring meals (this was most helpful after my in-laws left) and hire someone to clean if you can afford it so you have time to focus and adjust. And while the need for support is abundantly clear when your babies are born, it's true through the years too. Finding emotional support and connection through groups of moms, running groups, and even groups of running moms can be just as critical as tangible, everyday help, such as childcare.

LET GO OF REGRET

Mom guilt is a real thing, but the truth is, your kids will be far better off for having a parent who's strong, confident, and going after her goals. Often, we moms are hardest on ourselves, holding our thoughts and actions up to standards no human can (or should even strive to) achieve. Somehow, we think we should both go wholeheartedly after our own ambitions the same way we did before and be there for every moment of our kids' lives. It's just not practical, possible, or even desirable.

Of course, I feel these pangs and pressures too. Here are some of the things I found most helpful in coping with them.

Compartmentalize

Give all your attention to whatever you're doing at the present moment. When you're training, focus on being the best runner you can be; that way, when you're with your kids, you can flip completely to motherhood mode. You might have less time for each task, but if you do each with intention, you'll be more efficient and fulfilled.

See the Positive

Some situations have no upside, of course, but many hard choices can be viewed in a different light if you shift your perspective. For instance, after Rome was born, I felt guilty about sending Athens to preschool. I worked from home, I thought, so shouldn't I be able to watch them both? But then I realized it gave me special one-on-one time with Rome, which as a second child he wouldn't have otherwise. Meanwhile, Athens was really excited about this next step in his journey.

Prioritize Yourself

You can't pour from a cup that's empty. At this point, it's a cliché, but that doesn't make it any less true. If you don't build in time for a life of your own, you won't be nearly as good a mom, partner, friend, or person. (Oh yeah, and about the partner thing: It's always a good idea to build in dedicated time with your significant other too!) Doing something that fulfills us—whether that's running or another pursuit—truly allows us to be the parents we want to be when we're with our kids.

I know striking this elusive balance between who I am as a runner and a mom will be a lifelong work in progress. I can't wait to hear what's worked for other runner mamas out there too.

Grace, Without Pressure: Sara Vaughn

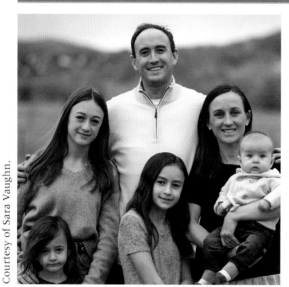

Courtesy of Sara Vaughn.

Sara Vaughn has juggled running and motherhood since her junior year at the University of Colorado. That's when she and her husband, Brent, who were teammates at the time, became parents to their first daughter, Kiki.

When Sara graduated in 2008, her priority was to go pro. "I felt like I needed to make money to justify the time I was committing to my sport," she says. "That put a lot of pressure on racing, and I found that I did not perform well that way."

Once she realized a big contract and the associated salary weren't in the cards for her, she charted her own course. She had a second daughter, Calia, then got her real estate license, aiming for a lucrative but flexible career. "Once I could provide for my family not based on running results, I did a lot better," she says.

Indeed, she seemed to get faster with each child. In August 2015, her third daughter, Cassidy, was born; 11 months later, she finished seventh in the 1,500 meters at the U.S. Olympic Trials. Then at the U.S. Championships in June 2017, when Cassidy was one, she ran a 61-second final lap to finish third in the same event. The performance earned her a trip to the 2017 IAAF World Track and Field Championships.

Now she has a fourth child—a son, Davey—and has fine-tuned the art of juggling a full-time job as a realtor, high-level training, and motherhood. "I schedule my runs, track sessions, and weight-lifting sessions as work appointments," she says. "I know nobody's paying me for those hours, but they make the rest of my day go much more smoothly if I schedule them in and prioritize." And, it continues to pay off—in 2021, she won her debut marathon, the California International Marathon, in 2:26:53.

Each return to the sport was a little more challenging physically, she says. But with experience also came wisdom. "What's nice is that I felt like I learned to give myself more and more grace with each pregnancy because I trusted myself more and more to 'come back,'" she says. "Our bodies are so amazing, especially if we treat them right and give them time."

Her biggest advice to other mother runners is to practice patience; seek expert help on preparing your pelvic floor for impact; and savor time with your family, even as you continue pursuing your goals. "Running can be a selfish endeavor. Even after I had kids, it's always something I wanted to do for myself," she says. "But more recently, I've included them in my goal-setting process. It's really interesting to hear what they think I can do. And the accomplishments that follow are so much sweeter."

FROM BARRIER TO BREAKTHROUGH

Remember, pregnancy and motherhood are far from the end of the line when it comes to your running goals. Patience, grace, and flexibility will get you through this time and on to even more meaningful breakthroughs on the other side. Here are some small, daily goals to get you through times when you're feeling stuck.

Barrier

I want to run during pregnancy, but fatigue or nausea is making it challenging.

Breakthrough Goals

Choose one or more.

I will do the following:

- Pinpoint a time in the day I feel best and run at that time
- Eat carbohydrate-rich snacks before, during, and after my run
- Head out for 5 or 10 minutes, knowing things may improve and if not, I can walk back home

---

Barrier

I can't run while pregnant, and it's breaking my heart.

Breakthrough Goals

Choose one or more.

I will do the following:

- Know I am enough, I'm doing the best thing for my baby, and my running goals will be there for me when I return
- Work with my doctor to find another safe way to move my body, for my mental well-being as much as my physical
- Add in another stress-relieving practice, such as yoga, meditation, or listening to calming music

Barrier

I want to come back to running postpartum; my doctor says I'm cleared, but I'm not sure where to start.

Breakthrough Goals

Choose one or more.

I will do the following:

- Start with short walks, then slowly add time as my body adjusts
- Keep the warning signs on page 79 in mind, and talk to my doctor if I experience them
- Seek out a postnatal core-training program, such as ReCORE
- Schedule appointments with a pelvic floor physical therapist or trained postnatal exercise specialist

---

Barrier

I find myself anxious or questioning my choices about running right now.

Breakthrough Goals

Choose one or more.

I will do the following:

- Find a mantra that resonates (Examples include "I make the best decisions for me and my baby" and "My body knows exactly what to do.")
- Seek support from other runner moms, a neighborhood group, or a close friend
- Carefully monitor my social media consumption, limiting it or muting accounts that make me feel jealous or unworthy

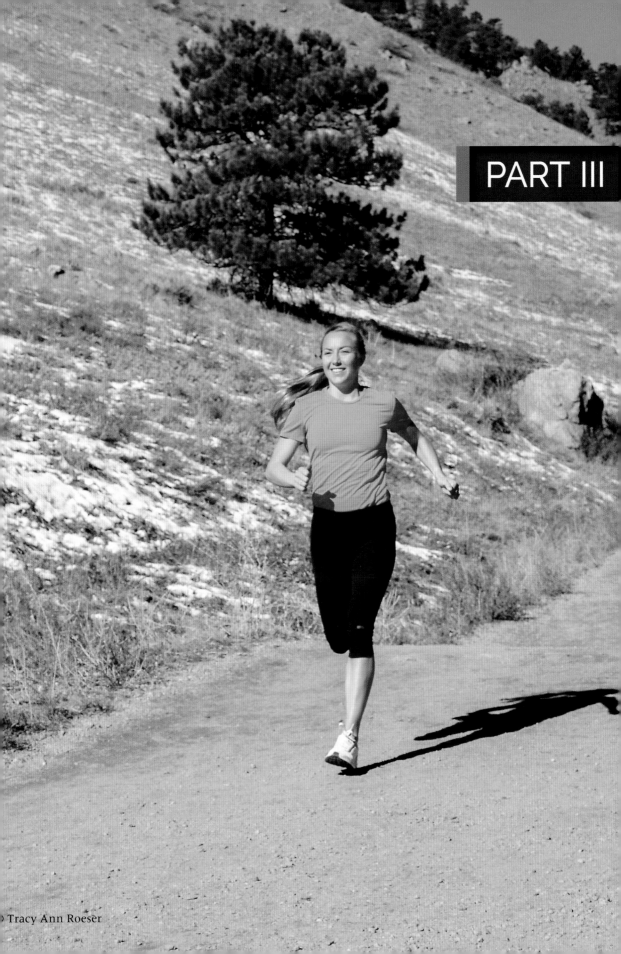

PART III

© Tracy Ann Roeser

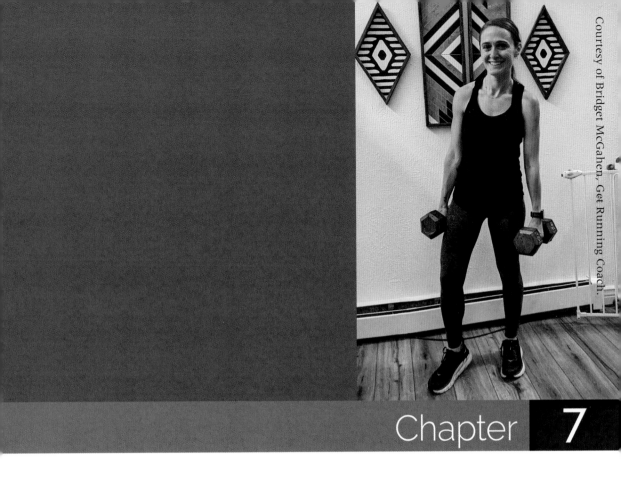

Chapter   7

Train Like an Athlete

"
As a coach and runner, I've seen too many athletes get injured running high mileage. As I implemented lower mileage and more strength, I've seen runners be able to get to the starting line not only healthy, but peaked.
"

Nell Rojas, coach, first American in the 2021 Boston Marathon, and Olympic Trials qualifier in the marathon and 10K

Yes, you have to run to reach your running goals, but you also have to think more broadly about preparing your body to perform your best. When used strategically, strength training and cross-training boost your fitness, protect you from injury, and keep your body and mind balanced and engaged.

As a runner, you probably know you *should* do these things, which we'll collectively call athletic training, but you might struggle with exactly how to fit them into a training schedule. It's not easy, especially when you're already balancing a busy life with big dreams. (As a mom and coach in addition to an elite runner, trust me—I get it!) With a little planning—and some quick but effective routines—you can transform yourself into a strong all-around athlete.

A STRONG FOUNDATION

Being the daughter of an Olympic marathoner definitely gave me some genetic advantages (and of course, my other parent is a 17:00 5K runner—thanks, Mom!). My dad, Steve Spence, also served as a built-in role model for hard work and a good attitude. And he gave me something else: the knowledge that there's more that goes into running fast than just more running.

In the 1980s, Poppa (as we call him) had already begun dabbling with strength training, something that wasn't common among endurance athletes at the time. The year I was born—1990—he began working with a strength coach named Doug Lentz, who overhauled his approach in the weight room. Soon, he was lifting heavy weights, doing fewer reps, and training his legs as well as his upper body in a program carefully coordinated with his training and racing schedule.

The results were remarkable, and the proof was shown in both an exercise science lab and his race results. He had more power in each step; a longer stride, which enabled him to cover more ground efficiently; and a lower injury rate. In fact, he believes this training was critical to his winning the 1992 Olympic Marathon Trials and making the U.S. team for the Barcelona Games.

When I started taking running seriously in eighth grade, I also began to lift in a way that made sense for my younger body. Doug owned a gym at the time, and eventually, I began working with him as well. Over the years, our families became good friends. I can even remember one Christmas Eve when the gym was closed, but our families got together there to lift anyway. I realize this is not a typical holiday in most households, but it was normal for us and so much fun!

I kept lifting through high school and college and into my professional running career. I've learned a lot from the strength coaches I've worked with and have reaped the benefits. Thanks to time spent in the gym, I've always been strong, coordinated, good at hills, and able to unleash a strong finishing kick at the end of races.

Cross-training, too, is something I've used since around age 13 to enhance my running. When I'm training hard, a weekly swim or aqua jog gives me an extra aerobic workout while the compression of the water refreshes my legs. During times when I couldn't run because of injury or pregnancy, the bike, pool, and elliptical offered opportunities to stay active and relieve stress, and each time I came back, they've been critical to rebuilding my fitness. Plus, it's just plain fun to break up the monotony of running sometimes and instead see the world from the pedals of a bike or elliptical outdoor bicycle.

Throughout my life, I've changed and adapted the ways I've approached athletic training, but I've never lost sight of the fact that when I use them with purpose, they make me a better runner. It starts with understanding how and why to incorporate them. From there, you can include them in a way that makes your entire training process effective, fun, and well matched to both your physiology and lifestyle.

LIFT TO LEVEL UP

As my family's experience shows, there are many good reasons to cross to the other side of the gym to the weight room or to carve out time at home for resistance exercises. Full-body strength training offers the following benefits:

- Builds durable muscles that can better absorb the impact of running so your body can handle more miles with less risk of injury
- Strengthens your bones (Hong 2019) (That's critical for women, especially as we age, to prevent conditions such as osteoporosis and fractures.)
- Fires up and strengthens the connections between your brain and your muscles, which allows you to run more efficiently, as physical therapist Jay Dicharry outlines in his book *Running Rewired* (Dicharry 2017)
- Improves your posture (That's especially important for moms who are constantly feeding, carrying, and rocking babies. Plus, it helps anyone who spends a lot of time hunched over a computer or phone, which is just about everyone these days.)
- Keeps your form from breaking down when you're tired at the end of a race or hard workout
- Evens out imbalances between your left and right sides, especially if you do single-leg exercises
- Addresses areas that are often weak in many women, especially moms (These areas include the muscles of the hips, pelvic floor, and glutes.)
- Fires up your body's fat-burning capabilities, which makes muscles leaner and more energy efficient (Vechetti et al. 2021)
- Boosts your balance, which is critical to running (After all, you're on one leg the entire time!)

All these benefits add up to two big, important perks for runners. First, per one research review and meta-analysis, strength training reduces your risk of injury by about one-third (Lauersen 2014).

Second, it makes you faster. According to results summarized in the *British Journal of Sports Medicine* in 2019, six months of strength training have been shown to improve performance in a time trial by 2 to 5 percent (Alexander 2019). That's about one to two minutes off your 10K time.

EVOLUTION OF AN ATHLETE

I suggest runners do strength moves two or three times per week. If you're new to this type of work, keep it simple. Start with a 5- to 15-minute routine with no equipment (try the core routine on page 95 or the body weight routine on page 96, doing one set of each exercise). From there, you have many options to progress your strength-training program. Here are a few ideas and guidelines to keep in mind.

Add On

As your body gets stronger, make the workout harder each week by adding additional reps and sets to each routine—but know that you don't have to spend hours at the gym. In fact, if you did, you'd risk overdoing it and interfering with your running progress. About 20 to 30 minutes will do the trick.

Branch Out

Try using equipment at home. Popular options include resistance bands, a physio ball, kettlebells, a suspension trainer, or dumbbells (see the resistance band routine on page 98 or the dumbbell routine on page 99). You can progress each of these routines by adding more sets and reps or by moving up to a higher weight or heavier resistance band.

Another option is a group exercise class, in person or online. Peloton and other apps offer strength-specific classes, as do some fitness studios. Barre classes, for instance, are primarily strength workouts. Other group options, such as Barry's Bootcamp and Orangetheory, blend strength training with a cardio workout (more on that in a bit).

Time It Right

Every four to six weeks, mix things up and try a new routine. That way, you keep things fun and strengthen different muscles in your core, upper body, and lower body.

Also, the week or two before a race, back off. Depending on your goals and plan, backing off could mean doing strength training fewer days, doing shorter workouts with fewer sets and reps or with lighter weights, or trading strength training for mobility routines. All these suggestions keep your muscles fired up and ready to go. Experiment and see what works best for you.

Get Help

Consider working with a personal trainer or strength coach. If you have the funds and access, expert guidance can be really helpful, even if it's only for a session or two. I strongly recommend a trainer or coach when you're moving up to heavier weights because form is crucial with a barbell or other free weights. Some coaches will work with you virtually or in pairs or small groups, which can be more affordable and still effective. Also, if you've been to a physical therapist after an injury, some of the exercises you were given might be worth keeping in your routine, even when you're healthy again, to prevent reinjury. Take that as an opportunity to ask a pro for a few basics that will keep your body in top form long after you've left the clinic.

Be a Strong Mama

Proceed with care during and after pregnancy. As we went over in chapter 6, your body is going through a lot in creating a new human. The types of exercises you can do will change as your baby grows and vary a lot from woman to woman. Always work with your health care team to know what's safe for you, and consider also consulting with a physical therapist or other pro who specializes in pelvic floor or other postpartum issues as you return to exercise after the baby is born.

STRENGTH BUILDERS

Heavy lifting and running can go hand in hand, but it's best to build up to that type of serious strength work under the guidance of a personal trainer or strength coach who has experience working with runners. Most runners can make significant progress with minimal equipment or even with body weight alone. Here are four routines to try. Even if you work your way up to three sets of each exercise, they'll still take you only about 20 minutes at the most.

Core Routine

Start with one to three sets of 10 repetitions of each move. As you improve, progress to 15 and eventually 20.

EXERCISE 1: MOUNTAIN CLIMBER

How it helps: Boosts your heart rate while working all your abdominal muscles

How to do it: Start in a high plank position with your hands directly under your shoulders. Engage your core by pulling your belly button in toward your spine. Bend your right knee in toward your right elbow. Then return it to the starting position; as you do, bring your left knee to your left elbow. Count one rep after each time both of your knees come forward. Continue, moving at a pace that feels right to you.

EXERCISE 2: ALTERNATING BIRD DOG

How it helps: Challenges your balance as your core works to stabilize the weight of your lifted arm and leg

How to do it: Start in a tabletop position. Raise your right leg straight out behind you, focusing on firing up your glute muscle. At the same time or slightly afterward, raise your left arm. Moving only your limbs, keep your back straight, core engaged, and hips square. Hold briefly, then return to the starting position. Repeat with your left leg and right arm for one rep.

EXERCISE 3: PLANK WITH SHOULDER TAP

How it helps: Continues working your core while adding a challenge to your arms, wrists, and shoulders

How to do it: Start in a high plank position or if needed drop to your knees. Keeping your core engaged and hips stable (again, you want as little movement as possible), lift your right hand and tap it against your left shoulder. Return to the starting position and repeat with your left hand on your right elbow for one rep.

EXERCISE 4: BICYCLE, FORWARD AND REVERSE

How it helps: Works your abs and obliques, the muscles along the sides of your waist

How to do it: Lying on your back, place your hands behind the back of your neck. Bend your knees 90 degrees and lift your legs until your shins are parallel to the floor. Then pretend to pedal a bicycle forward, starting by extending your right leg and bending your left. As your left knee bends, twist your upper body to the left, aiming your right elbow at your left knee. As your right leg bends, twist to your left for one rep. Keep your lower back pressed into the ground and repeat this movement continuously. After the desired number of reps, reverse the direction of the bicycle, moving your legs as if you were pedaling backward while continuing to twist toward your bent knee.

EXERCISE 5: GLUTE BRIDGE, ALTERNATING LEG LIFTS

How it helps: Strengthens those all-important butt muscles in addition to your abs and back

How to do it: Lie on your back with your arms at your sides, your knees bent, and your feet flat on the ground and hip-width apart. Drive through your heels to push your hips up, squeezing your glutes at the top (photo *a*). Keeping your hips up, lift your right leg (photo *b*) and lower it. Then lift and lower your left leg for one rep. Try to maintain as steady a bridge as possible, keeping your core and glutes engaged and moving only your legs.

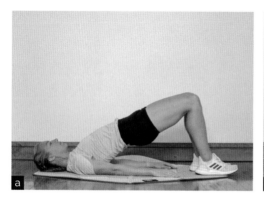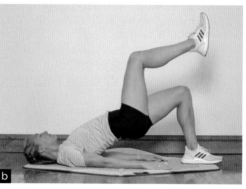

© Tracy Ann Roeser

(a) Glute bridge and *(b)* alternating leg lifts.

Body Weight Routine

Don't stress if you don't have a gym membership or any home equipment. You can do this routine, which works all the essential muscles of your legs and hips, with nothing but your own runner's body. Do one to three sets of 10 of each exercise.

EXERCISE 1: FORWARD LUNGE

How it helps: Strengthens your glutes, quads, hamstrings, hips, inner thighs, and core

How to do it: Stand with your feet hip-width apart. Engage your core, place your hands on your hips to stabilize them, and take a big step forward with your right leg. Lower until your right thigh is parallel to the floor. Your right knee might shift forward, but try not to let it wobble or extend over your right toe. Tap your left knee against the floor if you can, then press through your right heel to pop back up to standing. Repeat on the other side for one rep.

EXERCISE 2: CURTSY LUNGE

How it helps: Stabilizes your hips and strengthens your glutes

How to do it: Stand with your feet hip-width apart. Cross your right foot back behind your left and place it a foot or two beyond, staying up on your right toes (photo *a*). Then drop your right knee down until it's hovering just above the floor (photo *b*). Keep your hands on your hips and your eyes up so your back remains straight and tall; you should feel your left glute firing. Return to standing and repeat on the other side for one rep.

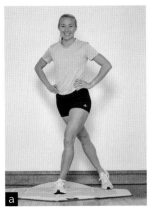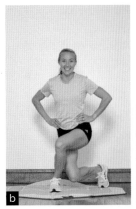

© Tracy Ann Roeser

Curtsy lunge *(a)* start and *(b)* finish.

EXERCISE 3: BACK LUNGE

How it helps: Strengthens your glutes, quads, hamstrings, hips, inner thighs, and core

How to do it: Stand with your feet hip-width apart. Engage your core and place your hands on your hips to stabilize them. Take a big step backward with your right leg, then lower until your left thigh is parallel to the floor and your right knee gently taps the floor. You'll feel this in the glute and quad of your left leg. Press through your left heel to pop back up to standing. Repeat on the other side for one rep.

EXERCISE 4: SQUAT

How it helps: Strengthens your legs and glutes

How to do it: Stand with your feet slightly wider than hip-width apart, your toes pointing slightly out and your arms straight out in front of you. Lower your butt down and back as if you were sitting in a chair. Pause briefly at the bottom, then return to standing, gently squeezing your glutes. Throughout the movement, keep your back straight, your eyes looking ahead, and your knees steady.

EXERCISE 5: SINGLE-LEG BALANCE WITH TRUNK ROTATION

How it helps: Improves stability while strengthening your legs and core, including your obliques

How to do it: Stand tall and lift your left leg until your thigh is parallel to the floor, your knee bent 90 degrees. Place your hands together at your chest (photo *a*). Rotate your trunk to the left over your bent knee and then back to center, staying balanced on one leg (photo *b*). It's OK if you wobble or have to touch your foot down briefly, but keep at it; running is just a series of single-leg balances, so stability in this position is huge! After the desired number of reps, repeat on the opposite side.

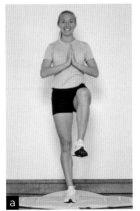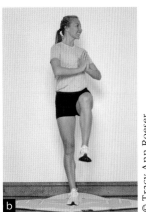

© Tracy Ann Roeser

Single-leg balance with trunk rotation *(a)* start and *(b)* finish.

Resistance Band Routine

If there's one piece of simple equipment to invest in, it's a set of resistance bands, which are small, elastic loops that come in different colors for different levels of challenge. They're inexpensive, portable, and incredibly effective in strengthening the muscles you need to run strong. I use TheraBand brand, but many others are available online and in running or sporting goods stores. Do one to three sets of 10 for each exercise.

EXERCISE 1: SUPERMAN

How it helps: Strengthens your core, back, and glutes

How to do it: Place the band around your ankles, then lie on your stomach, with your hands on the ground under your shoulders. Lift your upper and lower body at the same time, pushing out against the resistance of the band with your legs. Hold briefly at the top, then lower for one rep.

EXERCISE 2: MONSTER WALK, FORWARD AND BACKWARD

How it helps: Strengthens the muscles on the sides of your hips and glutes

How to do it: Stand up and place the band around your feet. Bend your knees slightly and stick your butt out, as if you were going to do a squat but go down only about a quarter of the way. Take a slow, controlled step forward with your right leg (photo) and then your left, for one rep. Keep the band tense; you should feel your glutes firing as you go. After 10 steps forward, reverse direction and take 10 steps backward.

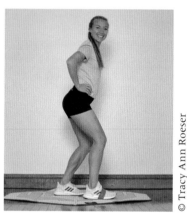

Monster walks

© Tracy Ann Roeser

EXERCISE 3: SKIER

How it helps: Strengthens glutes, hamstrings, and feet

How to do it: Stand with the band around your ankles with both knees slightly bent and your right hand on your hip, or touching lightly against the wall or the back of a sturdy chair if needed for balance. Completely extend your right leg behind you (photo). Then bend your right knee and move it forward again, without touching down if you can. After 10 reps, repeat on the other side.

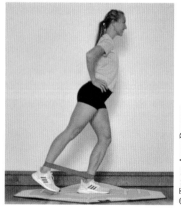

Skier

© Tracy Ann Roeser

EXERCISE 4: REVERSE CLAM

How it helps: Isolates your glutes, especially your gluteus medius, which stabilizes your hips when running

How to do it: Keep the band around your ankles and lie down on your left side with your hips stacked. Bend your hips and knees 90 degrees each—I call this the 90-90 (photo *a*). Lift your right leg slightly (photo *b*) and lower it back to starting—it's a small movement, but it won't take you long to feel the burn on the side of your right glute! After 10 reps, repeat on the other side.

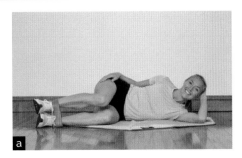

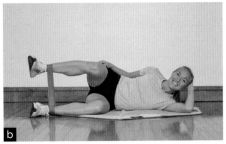

© Tracy Ann Roeser

Reverse clam *(a)* start and *(b)* finish.

EXERCISE 5: SIDE-LYING LEG LIFT

How it helps: Strengthens your glutes, hips, and obliques

How to do it: With the band around your ankles, lie on your left side again, but this time, keep your legs straight. Raise and lower your right leg, pulling it slightly back as you do while keeping everything else stable. Make sure your hips stay stacked and your right toe points slightly down. After 10 reps, repeat on the other side.

Dumbbell Routine

All you need for this workout is a set of two dumbbells—you'll want a weight that feels challenging, but not impossible—for one to three sets of 10 reps each (I'm using 10 pounds in these exercises). Whenever you're working with weights, it's important to stay focused and controlled so you don't get hurt.

EXERCISE 1: SPLIT SQUAT

How it helps: Strengthens quads, glutes, hamstrings, and core

How to do it: Stand with one dumbbell in each hand, then take a large step back with your right leg, as if you were doing a back lunge. Lower until your left thigh is parallel to the floor and your right knee taps against the floor, keeping the dumbbells down by your sides. Then push through your left heel to lift back up. After 10 pushes up and down, repeat on the other side.

EXERCISE 2: HAMMER CURL

How it helps: Strengthens biceps, core, and shoulders

How to do it: Stand with one dumbbell in each hand with your palms facing your body and your feet hip-width apart. Bend your right arm to bring the dumbbell up toward your shoulder. As you straighten and lower your right arm, bend your left arm and raise that dumbbell for one rep. Essentially, you're pumping your arms the same way you would when running, just with a little added resistance!

EXERCISE 3: GOBLET SQUAT

How it helps: Strengthens your entire posterior chain, including your hamstrings and glutes

How to do it: Stand with your feet slightly wider than hip-width apart with your toes pointing slightly out. Hold one dumbbell in both hands in front of your chest, gripping the top of it from underneath, as if you were holding a giant goblet. Lower back and down, as if you were sitting in a chair. Pause briefly at the bottom, then return to standing and gently squeeze your glutes. Keep the weight at chest level and your back straight with your eyes looking ahead and your knees steady.

EXERCISE 4: SINGLE-LEG RDL

How it helps: Strengthens your glutes and hamstrings and evens out imbalances

How to do it: Balance on your left leg and drive your right knee up 90 degrees with your right thigh parallel to the floor and right foot flexed. Hold a dumbbell in your right hand in front of your right thigh (photo *a*). Sit your hips back and keeping your back flat, bend at the waist until your right leg is straight behind you and the

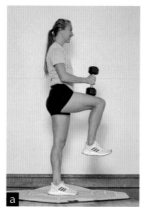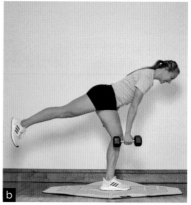

© Tracy Ann Roeser

Single-leg RDL *(a)* start and *(b)* finish.

dumbbell is about mid shin over your left leg (photo *b*). Don't stress about how far you go; it just depends on how flexible your hamstrings are. No matter what, you'll want to make sure you feel this in your left glute. (If you have trouble balancing, think about grounding through your left big toe.) Drive through your left heel and push your hips forward to return to the starting position. After 10 reps, repeat on the other side.

EXERCISE 5: SINGLE-LEG AND -ARM SHOULDER PRESS

How it helps: Works your hips, glutes, arms, shoulders, and obliques—one whole side of your body at a time

How to do it: Stand on your right leg and drive your left knee up in a running stance. Hold a dumbbell in your right hand, up next to the side of your face, with your elbow bent so the weight's at about your eye level (photo *a*). While balancing on your right leg, straighten your right arm to lift the weight above your head (photo *b*), then lower to the starting position. After 10 reps, repeat on the other side.

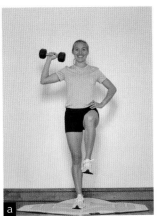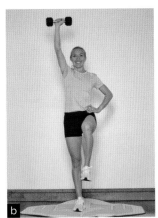

© Tracy Ann Roeser

Single-leg and -arm shoulder press *(a)* start and *(b)* finish.

CROSS PURPOSES

While strength training specifically builds stronger muscles, *cross-training* refers to other exercises that, like running, enhance your aerobic fitness. These workouts won't improve your running as much as running itself, but they can play a few important roles in your breakthrough. You can use cross-training for many purposes.

Build Fitness With Less Pounding

This can come in handy if you're injury prone. Some runners I coach replace a hard running workout with a hard cross-training session, such as an intense spinning or high-intensity interval class. That way, they are getting a really good challenge to their aerobic system with less risk of getting hurt. Others swap out an easy run for a more casual bike ride or a power walk.

Prevent—and Prepare for—Injury

Use cross-training to both prevent and prepare for injury. According to pro runner and coach Nell Rojas (see her profile on page 105), "Being able to feel comfortable backing off of running and having the skills to complete a high-quality cross-training workout is key to staying healthy." Having one or more types of cross-training integrated into your routine makes it easier to back off a bit when you develop a minor injury or to transition to cross-training alone when you're more seriously injured. As Nell says, "When a runner inevitably does get injured, having multiple cross-training methods is important so you don't get burned out on one and your body doesn't adapt to the other sport."

Stay Fit When You're Sidelined

Of course, even if you do everything right, you can still get hurt (more on this in chapter 8). When this happens, talk with your health care team about the types of exercises that are safe to do; from those, choose options that are convenient and fun for you. That second part is huge. If you hate getting wet or lack access to a deepwater pool, no one says you *have* to aqua jog, and forcing yourself to do so will only make you miserable. Try hiking or biking on a beautiful trail instead! Note that you won't be able to completely match the time, motion, or intensity of running with your cross-training—and that's OK. Your main goal here is to keep up the habit of training; boost blood flow to injured areas; and stay psychologically healthy, which is also crucial to your recovery.

Return to Running After a Break (or Create a Mini Break)

If you've been away for more than a week or two for any reason, especially injury or pregnancy, you will need to rebuild your mileage gradually. You can continue cross-training, ramping that down as you ramp up your running. For instance, after I had knee surgery in 2014, I started with an hour of low-resistance biking and moved on to the same amount of aqua jogging and then the elliptical. Once I started running on dry land—with two five-minute jogs—I would still get on the elliptical or bike for another 45 to 50 minutes. As my running time increased, my cross-training time decreased until I was running continuously. Cross-training also offers a small mental respite from running. Even when you're healthy, incorporating other activities you enjoy takes you out of the grind for a bit so your mood stays lifted and you truly enjoy the training process.

As we discussed in chapter 2, every run in your training plan has a purpose and so, too, should every cross-training workout. In the past, I've seen athletes fall into the "more is better" trap, trying to squeeze a quick bike ride or core session into every spare half hour. That often leads down the path to burnout and injury because your body will never have time to truly rest and recover. What's more, it can also be tied to disordered eating habits and a hyper-focus on weight that can interfere with your performance goals.

THE MYTHS—AND TRUTHS—OF ATHLETIC TRAINING

These common misconceptions pop up over and over again, but they're just plain wrong and can hold you back from your breakthrough. Here are the facts.

Myth: To get better at running, all you need to do is run.

Truth: While it's true you need to run to improve at running, athletic training has important benefits as well. It prepares your body to handle the miles you do log, prevents injury, and keeps you healthier and happier as a runner and human.

Myth: Strength training will make me too bulky to run well.

Truth: Any professional bodybuilder can tell you how much time, effort, and planning goes into sculpting extra-large, bulging muscles—not to mention all the careful meal planning. Two to three sessions of strength training per week might make your quads or biceps slightly more visible, but it's hardly going to add enough heft to negatively affect your speed. Remember, research suggests just the opposite—resistance training actually improves your performance.

Myth: Replacing a run with a cross-training session means you have to go two or three times longer.

Truth: Remember that every cross-training workout should have a purpose—and that's what should dictate how long you spend doing it. If you're swapping cross-training for an easy run, you can match up minute for minute, for instance, an hour-long bike ride for an hour-long run. If you're doing hard intervals in the pool or on the elliptical, that might take even less time than a running workout. With lower impact, your warm-up and rest periods can often be shorter.

Myth: If I cross-train during an injury, I can jump right back into mileage and workouts.

Truth: Cross-training while you're hurt, if it's not excessive, can preserve some of your fitness, not to mention your sanity. But because of the high impact of running, you'll still need to start gradually when you're coming back, or you'll risk a swift reinjury. Chapter 15 has a run-walk training plan that's perfect for this purpose.

CHOOSE YOUR ADVENTURE

There are many options for other types of cardio or aerobic workouts, such as pedaling, paddling, or pool running, that can complement your running. There's no single type of cross-training that's essential for all runners, so you should choose one or more that you like and are feasible based on your finances, location, and schedule. Table 7.1 covers a few upsides and downsides to consider for the most common types. Of course, there are many more options, from hiking to rock climbing to dance classes. Think creatively, though also carefully consider the risk of a fall, crash, or other injury as you focus on your running goals.

FITTING IT ALL IN

I hope by now you're sold on the benefits of athletic training, but you might be wondering when, exactly, you're supposed to do all this! The answer is going to be different for every runner. The training plans in chapters 12 through 15 can provide a starting point, but here are a few guidelines to keep in mind:

- Make hard days hard and easy days easy if possible. On the same day, I like to do my strength workouts after a hard workout or long run. That way, I can truly recover on my easy or rest days. Because you're probably doing your long run on the weekend, you likely have a little more time than you would on a weekday to fit in a quick 20- to 30-minute strength session afterward.

Table 7.1   Cross-Training Options

Mode	Pros	Cons
Aqua jogging	Replicates motion of running without impact; can aid recovery by compressive forces of water	Requires access to deep water; can be mentally challenging
Elliptical	Similar to running motion without impact; can be done at home or a gym or outdoors on an elliptical bicycle	Can be expensive or difficult to access; can be mentally challenging for long periods of time indoors (though music, podcasts, or streaming videos can be very helpful)
Indoor cycling	Has significant overlap with muscle groups used in running; good in any type of weather; can be done at home or a gym; can be fun because of competitive nature of a spin class	Can be expensive or difficult to access; can lead to going too hard on easy days because of competitive nature of a spin class
Outdoor cycling	Has some overlap with muscle groups used in running; provides psychological benefits of being in nature; allows more ground to be covered than running	Can be expensive or difficult to access; is weather dependent; presents risk of crashing
Rowing	Allows an intense full-body workout; is low impact	Can be expensive or difficult to access; is challenging to master form; has little overlap with running technique
Swimming	Is an extremely low-impact activity; can aid recovery by compressive forces of water; is beneficial for joint and muscle healing	Can be inconvenient to access; being in bathing suit not comfortable for everyone; has little overlap with running technique
Circuit or HIIT-style fitness classes, such as Barry's Bootcamp or Orangetheory	Usually combine strength training and cardio in one session; provide connection with a community; are often really fun	Can often be expensive; can interfere with recovery or increase risk of injury if too challenging; quality of guidance received highly dependent on instructor

- When that's not possible or you find it leaves you too wiped out, doing strength work the day before a hard workout is another good option. When I've tried this, I've found my muscles feel a bit more primed and ready for the running workout. Just make sure you schedule a rest or recovery day after those two days to make sure you don't overdo it.

- Cross-training can substitute for running on just about any day. Just be clear on the goal for that day's session, as mentioned in the Cross Purposes section on page 101. Treat cross-training intensity the same way you would running intensity; don't schedule an intense boot camp the day before or after a hard running workout, for instance.

So you see how all this can work together in a typical week, here's a template for a general schedule.

Monday	Easy run and core
Tuesday	Speed workout plus lifting
Wednesday	Spin class or aqua jog
Thursday	Tempo workout plus lifting
Friday	Easy run and core
Saturday	Long run
Sunday	Rest day

HIT THE MAT

You might have noticed that yoga and Pilates don't appear in either the strength-training section or the chart of cross-training modes on page 103. These movement types aren't as easy to categorize but can benefit your running and overall health in the following ways:

- Builds strength, especially in your core
- Enhances your mobility, increasing flexibility, and preventing injury (more on this in chapter 8, including some yoga-specific exercises starting on page 115)
- Links your breath to movement (discussed more in chapter 10)
- Offers a meditative aspect that improves mindset (more on that in chapter 9)
- Offers a little aerobic boost (as is the case with some power yoga classes)
- Offers convenience of being done at home with no or little equipment, though some types of Pilates classes involve a machine called a *reformer*

If you enjoy these workouts, you can use them in place of a strength, mobility, or cross-training session. As with other types of cross-training, however, you'll want to keep an eye on the intensity and how it might affect your running. Extremely vigorous or hot yoga classes can require some recovery time, so you might not want to do them the day before a long run or workout or when you're tapering for a race.

The Well-Rounded Athlete: Nell Rojas

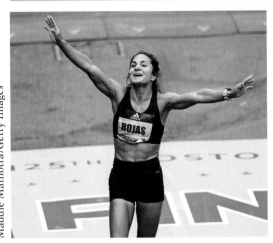

Nell Rojas is another athlete with an accomplished athlete as a father; her dad, Ric Rojas, set the 15K world record in 1981. Nell herself pursued an elite career in triathlon and obstacle course racing before narrowing her focus to running. Those sports involve a lot more than running, of course, and she believes the hours of athletic training she logged built a solid foundation of fitness and strength.

"I never felt good or performed well when running high mileage," Nell says, which, for an elite runner, means more than 90 miles a week. Many of the top female distance runners she competes against reach around 120 weekly miles. So as Nell prepared for her first marathon in 2018, the California International Marathon, she figured that meant she had about 30 miles per week to make up for with strength training, plyometric training, and cross-training.

Even with her background as an athlete and coach (she leads elite, adult, and youth running teams in Boulder and an online team called RISE in addition to owning a gym called The Speed Factory), she was still nervous heading into her first 26.2. "It's not the traditional way to train for a marathon, and I wasn't sure if I would have success," she says. On race day, she started out easy; picked up speed as she went; and finished with a 2:31:21, good enough to meet the Olympic Marathon Trials A standard. She took the same approach in training for Grandma's Marathon in 2019—and won, with a 2:28:06. And in 2021, she ran 2:27:12 to finish sixth—and first American—at the Boston Marathon.

Now confident in her approach, she works to instill confidence in her athletes. She recommends most of them run five or six days per week, cross-train one day, and strength train two days, with one day completely off.

Of course, the biggest challenge for those with jobs and families is finding the time, she acknowledges. She helps them fine-tune their schedules, getting the most out of every session. "There are times in the season where I tell them to prioritize their strength session over their run if they end up only having time for one, and times in the season where I tell them to do 20 minutes of their strength plan and a fraction of their run, and sometimes when I tell them to prioritize their run," she says.

Some athletes may see a temporary dip in their running times when they start strength training. For this reason, she recommends beginning early in their training cycle (preferably before the build-up for a big race), not in the final weeks of race preparation, and reassures athletes that as long as they put the same effort in, they'll reap the same rewards. After about six weeks, things typically start to click, with running times rebounding while power, strength, and durability rise.

"Even elite runners who have all day to prepare and recover from runs, have low daily stress, and make it their job to perform well and recover have a hard time staying healthy," she says. "So listen to your body and not the number of miles you think you should be running. Most importantly, keep yourself healthy so that you can run, because that's what brings us joy."

FROM BARRIER TO BREAKTHROUGH

You might identify most strongly as a runner, but it's time to claim the title of athlete. Small goals can help you begin this kind of training or fine-tune your approach once it's already a habit.

Barrier

I haven't cross-trained or strength trained regularly—or ever—and don't know how to start.

Breakthrough Goals

Choose one or more.

I will do the following:

- Today, as soon as I have time, do either the core routine or the body weight routine, then find one other day this week to repeat it
- Go over the list of cross-training activities and make a list of those that sound affordable, convenient, and fun

---

Barrier

I've dabbled in athletic training but don't know how to progress it to the next level or best use it to enhance my running.

Breakthrough Goals

Choose one or more.

I will do the following:

- Read over the section on progressing a strength program and pick one way to move forward in the next week, for instance, by increasing the number of sets and reps I'm already doing, using new equipment, or picking up a heavier band or weight
- Search and register for an online or in-person strength class that's appropriate for runners or sign up for one or two personal training sessions
- Write down a list of the types of cross-training I do, decide which purpose each one serves, and then look at my training schedule to see whether I need to make any adjustments in when and how I do them

Barrier

I have a hard time fitting athletic training into my schedule.

Breakthrough Goals

Choose one or more.

I will do the following:

- Look at my calendar and training schedule for the next month or this whole training cycle and slot in two 10- to 20-minute strength-training workouts per week (Note: Picking specific times, and even making them calendar appointments, can help them stick.)
- Cut back two of my runs by one or two miles and do strength work instead or just think about a day when I have time to run one extra mile and block in a short strength workout then
- For the next month, replace one easy run per week with a cross-training session of a similar length and intensity

---

Barrier

I really hate strength training and cross-training—all I want to do is run.

Breakthrough Goals

Choose one or more.

I will do the following:

- Reread the section on the benefits of athletic training and write down the sections that resonate with me so I can remind myself why it's important
- Try an online, app-based, or group fitness class that combines strength training and cross-training to maximize benefits
- Commit to trying one new strength routine and one new cross-training method each week until I find two or three I enjoy

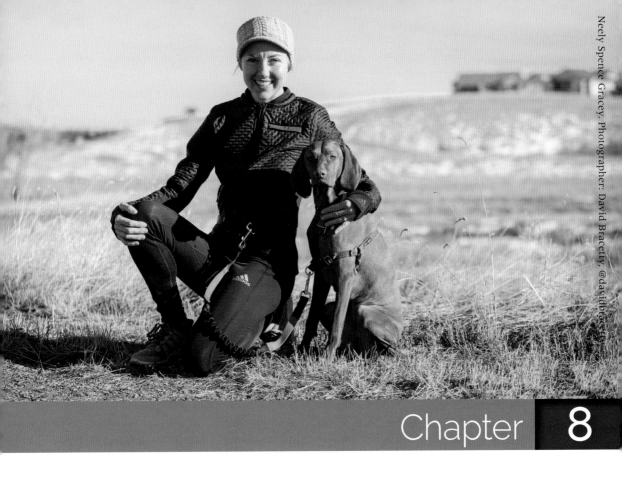

Neely Spence Gracey. Photographer: David Bracetty, @davidbracetty

Chapter **8**

Stay Healthy

❝ Injury, doubt, and anger have all been a part of my story. I'm trying to embrace all this and keep moving forward. Self-belief is huge for me, but it isn't always constant—and that's OK. Be brave and keep chasing your dreams. ❞

Emily Infeld, elite distance runner and Olympian

❝ A lot of times, athletes are so eager to make the event happen they don't take a step back. . . . I think trusting your team and trusting the process is instrumental in allowing athletes to overcome obstacles that can sometimes derail them from success. ❞

Dr. Heather Linden, director of physical therapy at UFC Performance Institute

Running is a high-impact sport, and most serious runners eventually deal with injuries. I've had plenty, from blisters to calf strains to a split kneecap. These setbacks are annoying at best and can feel devastating at worst.

But there are many ways to prevent injuries from happening in the first place as well as strategies to help you physically and mentally when they do pop up. With time and attention, you can build a set of routines to keep you healthy and strong, including actions targeting your individual weaknesses. And you can find a team of experts to help you thrive as a runner and a human.

THE UPS AND DOWNS OF INJURY

Nearly every runner has been there. You have a big goal in mind, a training schedule mapped out, and plenty of motivation to make it happen. Then suddenly, your knees begin aching, your calf pops, or slight soreness in your foot increases until you can barely walk.

Believe me when I say I understand both the sinking feeling that sets in and the temptation to ignore or downplay pain. In 2017, I had swelling in my foot while preparing for the New York City Marathon. Had I taken a week off when it started, I probably could have saved my season. But I wanted to race in July and August, so I kept pushing through. After the Falmouth Road Race, it hurt so badly that I couldn't even cool down, forcing me to take the week off. It wasn't long enough, and I had to withdraw from New York to rest.

However, I've also experienced the flip side. Often, if you catch an injury early, have a plan for coping with it, and stay flexible with yourself and your training, you can still proceed with your plans.

Take my previous training cycle for New York in 2016. I ran the Staten Island Half Marathon three weeks before. I won the race, but the weather was rainy, cold, and windy, and I had to catch a four-hour flight back home soon after.

My calves tightened up right away. I got a massage, and they felt a little better. But then, on an easy run a few days later, my right calf completely seized, and I had to walk—or really, limp—home. Immediately, I felt my dreams of finishing in Central Park slipping through my fingers.

After a minor freak out, I refocused. I went to see a physical therapist, Dr. Heather Linden, who then was at the Colorado Springs Olympic Training Center. She reassured me that if we did everything right, I could make it to the race. I trusted her and was willing to follow her guidance to make it happen.

The plan included taking four complete days off and skipping my last 22-mile-long run. Dr. Linden did lots of dry needling, cupping, and mobility work on my leg. The following week, I moved most of my mileage onto an antigravity treadmill, including a 19-mile-long run.

Instead of fretting about not being outside, I took the opportunity to watch a video of the marathon course, practice my fluid and fuel intake, and even adjust the grade of the treadmill for all those bridges and hills. I didn't finish an entire run outside again until October 27. But on race day, November 6, I still felt great and set a new personal best of 2:34.

Now, as a professional athlete whose job it is to perform well, I had advantages not available to everyone. You might not be able to see a physical therapist every day or run on a high-tech treadmill. But the key lesson I took from this experience applies to anyone: all the training I'd put in before the injury mattered far more than a few days off and missing a long run. Adjusting, instead of pushing through, made it possible for me to line up and run a PR.

Over my career as an athlete and a coach, I've learned from both my successes and mistakes. I now know smart athletes take a three-step approach to injury. First, they nail the basics, taking active steps to prevent getting hurt in the first place. Then they tune in to their bodies and make adjustments to address small things before they get bigger. Finally, they plan for the worst by knowing what they'll do when aches and pains don't go away or a full-blown injury develops despite their best efforts.

STEP ONE: NAIL THE BASICS

Just like a good training program starts with building a base, a smart injury-prevention strategy begins with a solid foundation. We get deeper into each of these areas in other chapters, but here's a quick overview:

- *Prioritize rest (chapter 3).* When you're working hard in training, your body needs lots of downtime to adapt and become fitter and stronger. This is why athletes build in rest and recovery days when they're either running very easy or not running at all.
- *Get enough sleep (chapter 3).* Sleep is when your body repairs and rebuilds. Experts generally agree healthy adults need seven to nine hours (Watson et al. 2015), but you might need more than usual when you're training hard.
- *Eat enough, especially of whole, nutritious, and anti-inflammatory foods (chapter 4).* Underfueling increases your risk of any type of injury, especially bone injuries. Some critical nutrients include protein, iron, calcium, magnesium, and vitamin D.
- *Keep your training well rounded (chapter 7).* Strength training and cross-training increase your resilience. Plus, if you already have cross training in your routine, it's way easier to swap a bike or swimming workout for a run when you need a little break.
- *Work on your mindset (chapter 9).* The same types of mental skills that enable you to handle tough training—such as managing stress and using positive self talk—can reduce your risk of injury and help you cope if it happens.

STEP TWO: TUNE IN

Once you have the basics down, it's time to go to the next level. You've probably heard the phrase "listen to your body." It's a simple enough concept but sometimes hard to know how to put into practice.

And honestly, it's not the full picture. Not only do you need to hear the messages your muscles, joints, and tendons are sending you, but you also need to know what to do in response. It's really a two-way conversation!

Here's how I approach it myself and with the athletes I coach:

- *Know your weaknesses.* Complete an injury history and assess your lifestyle to identify your vulnerabilities so you can take steps to balance them.
- *Monitor your status.* Do regular mobility work. During these exercises—and your runs—note whether something feels tighter or sorer than usual or one side's different than the other.
- *Make small tweaks.* Address small twinges or imbalances by changing your training, adding extra mobility moves, or using home treatments (see At-Home Tools, page 113, and Build Your Own Routine, page 120).
- *Follow the three-day rule.* If a surprising new ache or pain pops up or something small bothers you for three days in a row, I recommend first trying three days off. The body's inflammatory response takes about 72 hours to resolve minor issues,

so often, that's all you need. I remember once having a sudden pain on the top of my foot; I thought it might even be a stress fracture! But after three days of rest, ice, and anti-inflammatory medications (I usually take naproxen and curcumin, a natural remedy, but check with your health care team on this), it felt completely fine.

- *Watch for red flags.* Some signals mean *stop*. Runners should never train through a broken bone or stress fracture, says Dr. Linden (now the director of physical therapy for the UFC Performance Institute). Also, stop and seek medical attention if you have severe bruising and swelling, your symptoms don't improve within 48 hours, or you aren't able to bear weight without pain.

Know Your History

When I start working with new coaching clients, I ask them to complete an injury history. Study after study finds that getting hurt once increases your chances of it happening again (Dallinga et al. 2019; Van Poppel et al. 2018). My job as a coach is to help athletes break this cycle.

Sometimes, runners will report major injuries—for instance, a knee surgery a few years ago—from which they're fully recovered. They'll also tell me about ongoing issues, such as intermittent hamstring tightness, a sore back that's fine as long as they visit the chiropractor regularly, or tightness in the IT (iliotibial) band unless they're diligent about foam rolling and hip strengthening.

Take some time to put together your own injury history—write it down or type it up. Include treatments you've tried at home or through a professional (especially if they helped). Keep this information handy so you have a plan if and when the same thing crops up again. And take it with you to injury-related medical appointments—a complete picture makes it easier for health care providers to diagnose and treat you.

Assess Your Risk

A few lifestyle factors may influence your injury risk. Table 8.1 describes some of the issues I look for in my athletes and how I suggest they approach them.

Track Your Pain

As mentioned, it's helpful to record any tight spots or minor aches in your training log. I use a paper log, but you can also do this in your GPS app, Strava, or wherever you keep track of your training. I often make notes such as "left calf sore at the end of the run," "right knee achy on the downhills," or "right arch tight for the first mile." (Final Surge, which is the log I use with my coaching clients, offers a specific spot to report it, including a sketch where you can pinpoint exactly where on your body the problem is.)

With notes, I can see how long an issue sticks around and spot trends and potential solutions. For instance, if my left calf is sore after three hill workouts in a row, going up or down seems to be causing a problem. To address it, I might skip hill repeats for a week or two, adjust my form, or take a few extra minutes to roll out my calves before I tackle hills the next time.

Taking note of your mood during and after each run can help too. Sometimes, when my clients have a string of bad workouts or negative emotions, they're related to life stress or weather conditions, but in other cases, they're actually a warning sign of an impending injury. Resting a few days when you're just not feeling it can give your body time to heal things before they even hurt and your mind some time to relax and recharge.

Table 8.1   Balance Your Odds

Issue	Effects	How to offset the effects
Long hours at a desk job	Extended sitting tightens muscles and tendons, such as your hip flexors, making them prone to extra strain.	Take frequent breaks throughout the day, use a standing desk to alternate positions, and do a dynamic warm-up before each run to stretch hip flexors and activate glutes.
A job that keeps you on your feet all the time, such as teaching or nursing (especially if you work a night shift)	Your body has less time and energy for recovery because night shifts disrupt sleep.	Plan hard workouts around long shifts, coordinate races around yearly schedules (teachers can often train hard in the summer and race well in early fall), and allow plenty of time to increase mileage and achieve your goals.
Stressful life periods	High cortisol levels increase your risk of injury and reduce your body's ability to recover from hard training (Singh and Conroy 2017).	Back off your training, add in stress relievers (see chapter 9), and readjust your timelines or your goals.
Other medical issues	A history of eating disorders can increase the fragility of athletes' bones; other diseases or treatments for them can also contribute to injuries.	Consult your health care team about the best way to train safely, stay on top of ongoing treatments, take extra rest days when you're sick or fatigued, and allow plenty of time to increase mileage and achieve your goals.
Recent childbirth	Postpartum, you may have diastasis recti—a separation of your abdominal muscles—or weak pelvic floor muscles.	See a pelvic floor physical therapist, focus on appropriate core exercises (more in chapters 6 and 7), and allow plenty of time to increase mileage and achieve your goals.

At-Home Tools

Some treatments that prevent and treat injuries (think acupuncture or dry needling) are limited to a medical office. However, there are more tools than ever that you can use at home to relieve pain and promote healing.

Things can get a bit tricky here because there's not always a lot of scientific evidence about exactly how or in what situations these methods work. I've found my own favorites by following advice from my treatment team and through trial and error.

While some might cause discomfort (foam roller, I'm looking at you!), you should stop if you feel serious or unexpected pain, or they seem to make an injury worse. Always ask a sports medicine professional if you have questions or concerns.

Here are a few of my go-tos:

- Rollers, for releasing tension and increasing mobility
- Lacrosse ball or tennis ball, for more targeted self-massage
- Massage guns, especially those that provide a percussive, deeper muscle treatment
- Resistance bands for strength and mobility work
- Scrapers, to break up adhesions in hard-working muscles (I also use a regular old spoon for this purpose!)
- Bone healing stimulator, which uses ultrasound waves to boost bone repair and rebuilding
- Kinesiology tape, which offers pain relief and support for muscles, tendons, and ligaments
- Ice baths and ice packs, for reducing swelling and inflammation

- Hot pads and hot baths, which relax tight muscles (You can also alternate them with cold for a contrast treatment that boosts blood flow.)
- Home cupping set, which I use to relieve soreness and tension, especially in my calves, IT band, and back
- A treadmill attachment from LEVER that allows you to take up to 45 pounds off your body weight

Mobility Moves

Mobility exercises loosen your body, balance your muscles, and pinpoint areas that are sore, tight, and in need of additional attention. I have an entire 20-minute mobility routine I do two or three times a week, before or after a long run or workout (you can find the whole thing on my YouTube channel). Here are some of my favorite exercises, and table 8.2 lists a few ways to combine them. For exercises with the foam roller or lacrosse ball, pause on any particularly sore or tight spots, then breathe deeply and feel them gently release.

Table 8.2   Targeted Training

Problem	Exercises
Tight hips	• Hip flexor stretch into TFL (tensor fasciae latae) roll • Groiner • Three-part lunge • Iron cross • Scorpion
Tight or sore lower back	• Cat-cow • Child's pose to cobra • Mermaid • Downward dog series • Foam roll back
Tight or sore shoulders	• Shoulder circle with band • Rolling back to shoulders • Cat-cow • Child's pose to cobra • Mermaid
Knee pain or stiffness	• IT band to hip to quad roll • Side-lying quad stretch • Glute bridge • Clamshell • Downward dog series part 1, walk the dog
Tightness or soreness in the calf, shin, or foot, including pain from plantar fasciitis, an inflammation on the bottom of the foot	• Foot and arch roll • Calf roll • Downward dog series • Heel drop • Toe lift
Full-body mobility	• Three-part lunge • Foam roll back • Shoulder circle with band • IT band to hip to quad roll • Heel drop

EXERCISE 1: HIP FLEXOR STRETCH INTO TFL ROLL

How it helps: Opens up hips, helps prevent side stitches

How to do it: Lie on your back with your upper back and head resting on the floor and the foam roller under your hips (photo *a*). As you feel your hips release, lightly massage the front of your hips and obliques with your hands. After about 15 to 20 seconds, bend your left knee and twist your lower body to your right side; for about 10 seconds, gently roll the TFL, a key muscle on the side of your hip (photo *b*). Return to the starting position, then repeat on the other side, bending your right knee and twisting to your left.

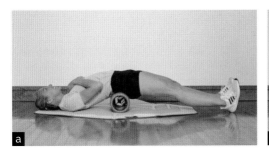 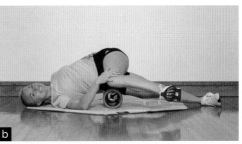

Hip flexor stretch into TFL roll *(a)* start and *(b)* finish.

EXERCISE 2: THREE-PART LUNGE

How it helps: Stretches hip flexors and obliques

How to do it: Kneel down, then step your left foot forward, bending your knee at a 90-degree angle. Hold the foam roller in front of you with your arms outstretched. First, pulse forward gently with your hips as you lift the roller over your head (photo *a*). Repeat five times. Then extend your torso to lift the roller above your head and to your left while again gently pulsing forward five times (photo *b*). Finally, hold the roller out in front of you again and fully twist your torso to your right five times, over your planted knee, and keep the roller level (photo *c*). Switch your legs and repeat all three movements on the other side.

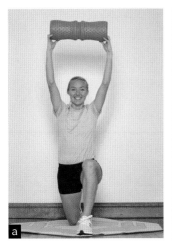 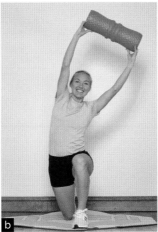 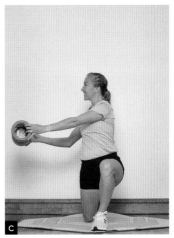

Three-part lunge *(a)* start, *(b)* middle, and *(c)* finish.

EXERCISE 3: GROINER

How it helps: Opens up hips, activates core

How to do it: Start in a high plank position. Engage your core; bend your right knee; and draw your right foot forward, placing it down by your right palm. Lower your left knee toward the ground and feel the stretch along the front of your left hip as you look forward. Hold for one second, return to the starting position, and repeat on your left side. Repeat five times on each side.

EXERCISE 4: IRON CROSS

How it helps: Opens hips, chest, and back

How to do it: Lie on your back with your arms stretched out like a "T." Keeping your upper body still, kick your right leg across your body, aiming to touch your right toe to the floor approximately level with your waist (photo *a*). Return to center, then repeat with your left leg kicking to your right side (photo *b*). Repeat five times per leg.

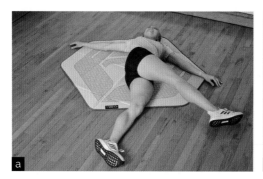
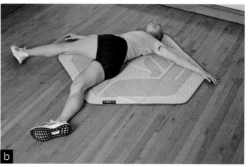

Iron cross *(a)* start and *(b)* finish.

© Tracy Ann Roeser

EXERCISE 5: SCORPION

How it helps: Opens hips, chest, and back

How to do it: Lie on your stomach with your arms stretched out like a "T." Keeping your upper body still, kick your left leg across your body to your right, aiming to touch your left toe to the floor approximately level with your waist (photo *a*). Return to center, then repeat with your right leg kicking to your left (photo *b*). Repeat five times per leg.

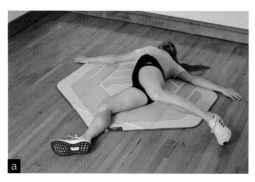
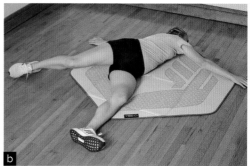

Scorpion *(a)* start and *(b)* finish.

© Tracy Ann Roeser

EXERCISE 6: CHILD'S POSE TO COBRA

How it helps: Opens the shoulders and back, activates core

How to do it: Start in child's pose—kneel down and lower your torso toward the floor, stretching your arms out in front of you as you ease your hips back toward your heels. On an inhale, pull your shoulders back and push your chest forward; lower your hips toward the ground; and straighten your legs, leaving your toes pointed. You'll feel a nice stretch in your chest as your back bends. Exhale to return to child's pose. Repeat five times.

EXERCISE 7: DOWNWARD DOG SERIES

How it helps: Stretches calves and shoulders

How to do it: Begin in downward dog pose (photo *a*)—place your palms on the ground beneath your shoulders with your feet about shoulder-width apart, your heels as close to the floor as possible, and your hips raised.

- Walking the dog: Lower one heel while raising the other, five times on each side (photo *b*).

- Double heel raise: Lift up on the tiptoes of both feet five times (photo *c*).

- Shoulder press: Gently pulse your head, chest, and shoulders down (not pictured).

- Three-legged dog: Kick your right leg back and up (photo *d*), then bring your right knee forward toward your right elbow (photo *e*). Repeat five times, then switch legs and repeat five more times with your left leg.

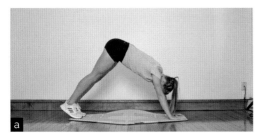
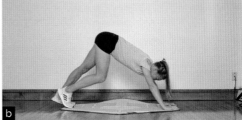
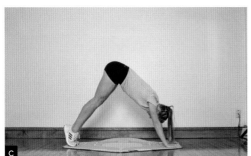
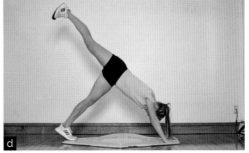
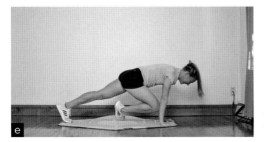

© Tracy Ann Roeser

Downward dog series *(a)* beginning, *(b)* walking the dog, *(c)* double heel raise, *(d, e)*, three-legged dog.

EXERCISE 8: CAT-COW

How it helps: Activates and opens up back and core, aligning breath with movement

How to do it: Kneel on the floor in tabletop position and place your hands on the foam roller or the floor. Take a big breath in. On the exhale, tuck your chin and arch your back up like a cat. Inhale again, moving to cow—look up, drop your back and stomach down, and stick out your butt. Repeat five times.

EXERCISE 9: MERMAID

How it helps: Stretches obliques, mobilizes back

How to do it: Sit with both your legs folded so the knees point to your left side, making sure the inside of your right foot is flat against the ground. Reach your right arm up and bend over toward your left, lowering your left arm toward the ground and feeling a stretch down your right side. Return to start, then reach to the other side; repeat five times. Then switch sides, folding your legs to your right and reaching five times again.

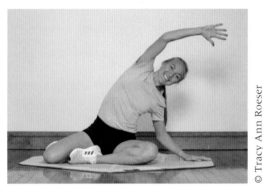

Mermaid.

© Tracy Ann Roeser

EXERCISE 10: FOAM ROLL BACK

How it helps: Opens up chest, shoulders, and obliques; releases thoracic spine

How to do it: Lie on your back with the foam roller underneath your shoulders. Place your hands behind your head, bend your knees, and roll slightly up toward your neck, then all the way down to your tailbone. After 20 to 30 seconds, twist your upper body to your right and left for about 5 to 10 seconds each side to gently massage your obliques.

EXERCISE 11: SHOULDER CIRCLE WITH BAND

How it helps: Opens up shoulders and chest

How to do it: Kneel down and hold a light resistance band in both hands, starting with your palms down and your arms by your sides. Keeping your arms straight, circle them overhead and behind your back, feeling the tension in the band. Circle your arms back overhead and to your front to return to the starting position. Repeat 10 times. (If you don't have a band or it's too challenging, large arm circles accomplish the same goal.)

EXERCISE 12: ROLLING BACK TO SHOULDERS

How it helps: Releases tension and stiffness in the back and shoulders

How to do it: Lie on your back and place a lacrosse ball under the base of your right shoulder blade, near your spine. (If the lacrosse ball is too hard, you can use a tennis ball instead.) Raise your right arm over your head and wiggle side to side and up, working the ball toward the top of your shoulder. If you want to add pressure or change the angle, lift your hips and back off the ground. After 30 seconds (or longer if you'd like), repeat on your left side.

EXERCISE 13: IT BAND TO HIP TO QUAD ROLL

How it helps: Loosens the sides of the hips and the quads, which may relieve hip and knee pain

How to do it: Lie on your right side with your right arm on the floor and the foam roller under your right hip. Using your body weight as leverage, roll from your hip down, stopping before your knee. After about 15 seconds, rotate so both hands and your left knee rest on the ground, rolling out your right quad and the front of your right hip. Next, move to your left quad, then twist to the side to roll out your left hip.

EXERCISE 14: SIDE-LYING QUAD STRETCH

How it helps: Stretches the quads and hips

How to do it: Lie on your left side; bend your right knee and reach back to grab your right ankle with your right hand. Kick your leg backward while pulling gently with your hand—you'll feel the stretch in your quad. Repeat five times, then flip to your right side, grab your left ankle with your left hand, and do five more.

EXERCISE 15: GLUTE BRIDGE

How it helps: Activates glutes

How to do it: Lie on your back with your knees bent and your feet flat on the floor. Push your hips up until they form a straight line with your knees and shoulders. Keep your core engaged and squeeze your glutes, especially at the top. Lower to the floor, then repeat five times.

EXERCISE 16: CLAMSHELL

How it helps: Activates and strengthens hips

How to do it: Lie on your left side with your knees bent and your legs stacked on top of each other. Engage your core and, keeping your feet together and your hips and pelvis still, raise your right knee—essentially opening your legs like a clamshell. Return to the starting position, then repeat five times. Add a mini band above your knees for an additional challenge.

EXERCISE 17: FOOT AND ARCH ROLL

How it helps: Releases tension in the arch and ball of the foot

How to do it: Stand up and place a lacrosse ball under the base of your right toes. (If you need to, you can hold on to a wall or something else stable for balance, and if the lacrosse ball is too hard, you can use a tennis ball instead.) Roll the ball around across the width of your foot and then back and forth across the arch, massaging the whole bottom of your sole. After 30 seconds (or longer if you'd like), repeat on your left side.

EXERCISE 18: CALF ROLL

How it helps: Releases tension in the calves and shins

How to do it: Sit up with your hands on the floor behind you. Bend your left knee and place your left foot on the floor, then the foam roller under your right calf. Raise your hips and roll back and forth along your calf; as you do, rotate your lower right leg, and point and flex your toes to target different areas of the soleus and gastrocnemius muscles that make up your calf. After about 30 seconds, repeat on your left leg.

EXERCISE 19: HEEL DROP

How it helps: Stretches and strengthens calves and feet

How to do it: Stand with your right foot on a step or bench with your heel hovering off the edge. Hold onto the wall or something else stable for support. Lower your right heel slowly, feeling the stretch in your calf. If you keep your right leg straight, you'll stretch your gastrocnemius, the large, two-part muscle that makes up the bulk of your calf; if you bend your knee, you'll stretch your soleus, the deeper calf muscle. Push up with one or both of your legs to return to the starting position, then repeat five times before switching legs.

EXERCISE 20: TOE LIFT

How it helps: Mobilizes and strengthens the feet

How to do it: Sit in a chair or on the floor with your knees bent and your feet flat on the floor. Keeping your four little toes still, lift your right big toe, then push it down into the floor. Repeat five times. Then keeping your big toe still, lift and press your four little toes. Repeat five times, then repeat both movements on your left foot.

Build Your Own Routine

By combining advice from medical professionals, tips from other runners and coaches, and a little self-experimentation, you can design your own plan for addressing common issues. Since pregnancy, I've dealt on and off with shin splints. I spent months trying to figure out why I was getting them and how to get rid of them.

Now, when I feel my shins start to tighten, I do the following:

- Foam roll my calves to identify tight spots, then continue loosening them up with the R8 deep-tissue massager (I also roll my feet on the R3.)
- Stretch my calves on the stairs—once with bent knees and once with straight knees, holding 30 seconds each time (see Heel Drop)
- Use my home cupping set to release tight fascia (With the set I have, flushed skin indicates I'm in the right spot.)
- Scrape along remaining, stubborn tight spots with a spoon
- Freeze a small paper cup full of water, then take it out and rub it on my shins for a DIY ice massage

This routine takes me 30 to 45 minutes, depending on how tight or sore I am. Once I'm done, I put on shoes to take a little pressure off my calves and try to rest my legs for the rest of the day. I'm typically back to normal within a day or two. And if I'm not—well, I know it's time to get an expert involved.

This exact plan might not work for you, or you might have a different problem area (or less time in your day to work on it). But when you develop strategies like these, an ache or pain becomes an issue you can proactively address, rather than a devastating blow to your progress. In other words, it's as good for your mindset as it is for your muscles.

STEP THREE: PLAN FOR THE WORST

No matter how many precautions you take, you will probably end up sidelined with an injury at some point. Sometimes, it's sudden—let's say you fall and tear a tendon or break a bone. In other cases, a small niggle turns into a pain you can't ignore, even after you try rest and home treatments.

I won't lie and tell you it's not a huge bummer to be injured. But I will say that acknowledging that it may happen—and having a plan for how to handle it—can make the process suck a lot less. Here are the steps I recommend taking.

Be Upset

You might be surprised to hear this. After all, shouldn't you put your injury in perspective because time off from running isn't the worst problem you could have? Sure, but if you're invested enough in your training to set big goals and aim for them, running means a lot to you. You should feel frustrated and sad when you have to stop, and you should honor your commitment and emotions by giving yourself at least a day or two to wallow in the disappointment. In fact, doing so gives you the best odds of coming back stronger, according to a study by British sport psychology researchers (Salim and Wadey 2018).

Then Move Forward

Don't stay down in the dumps. Once you've processed what's happened—maybe by journaling (more on that in chapter 9) or talking it out with a running buddy or a sport psychologist—let go of negative emotions and take action. Until you're back to full training again, treat recovery as your sport, recommends Carrie Jackson, a certified mental performance consultant (and Cindy's coauthor on *Rebound: Train Your Brain to Bounce Back Stronger from Sports Injuries*). Pour all the time and dedication you were putting into your training into steps such as consulting a medical professional for a diagnosis, sticking to a treatment plan, and working on your mental skills. And you can also consult a mental skills coach or a sport psychologist to help you get through this part of the process. Your mental health is as important as your physical health—and injury can bring on bouts of depression, anxiety, and other negative emotions, especially if you've had a history of them.

Revisit Your Goals and Timeline

We'll talk more about dealing with setbacks in chapter 16. In most cases, injuries aren't barriers to your breakthrough but rather important steps along the way. If taking time to heal an injury means you have to choose a different race to target (or if not possible, adjust your time goal), you haven't failed. It's all part of the journey of this tough but beautiful sport.

GO TO THE PROS

Every serious runner can benefit from building a trusted team of professionals who understand the athlete's body. Some of these professionals might be people you visit regularly to ward off injury, whereas others are the type you'll call when something flares up. (And some of them are superheroes who can handle it all!)

The types of people you may want on your team include the following:

- Chiropractors (Those who use the initials DACBSP or CCSP have completed additional training in sports medicine and are certified through the American Chiropractic Board of Sports Practitioners.)
- Physical therapists
- Massage therapists
- Athletic trainers

- Podiatrists
- Complementary or holistic providers, such as acupuncturists and naturopathic doctors
- Orthopedic doctors (Look for those who are members of the American Orthopaedic Society for Sports Medicine. Some are surgeons, and others specialize in nonsurgical treatment. Ask which one you're seeing when you make or go in for an appointment.)

Often, athletes will go to a doctor who is close by or they found online—but that person may not be the most qualified to work with dedicated athletes, Dr. Linden points out. Your baseline and goals as an athlete differ from those of someone who doesn't run regularly. Don't be afraid to be straightforward about your needs, to ask lots of questions, or to get a second opinion if you're not happy with how you're progressing or a doctor recommends an aggressive treatment, such as surgery, Dr. Linden says.

As a pro runner near Boulder, Colorado, I'm lucky to have lots of qualified medical professionals nearby. It might not be so easy to find them in other places! But no matter where you are, there are a few ways to find these experts:

- Ask other athletes for referrals
- Call or search online to find out which professionals treat athletes at your local university or on pro sports teams or handle medical services for races
- Take advantage of injury screenings or professional consultations at race expos, running stores, and group runs (Bonus: You can often get free, expert advice and possibly a group discount on future services.)

I also want to acknowledge other obstacles, such as insurance coverage and financial resources. If you have an HMO, for instance, you might have to first see a primary care doctor for a referral. Some of these services may not be covered at all. (If you're fortunate enough to have a choice about your coverage plan, keep this in mind—sometimes, a few extra dollars a month in premiums can save you big bucks in copayments or out-of-network charges later on when you're managing an injury.)

If you don't have coverage for a specific service, inquire about payment plans, reduced rates for self-paying patients, or sliding-scale fees. Surprisingly, many types of providers can and will negotiate if you ask.

Note that it's also a great idea to find doctors who have experience with athletes for all your medical needs. If your primary care doctor, ob-gyn, or dermatologist is a runner or at least understands runners, you're far more likely to get advice, testing, and treatment that meshes with your lifestyle. For instance, Dr. Linden points out that an EKG or ECG of an athlete's heart will read very differently than the results of the same test from someone who is not regularly active.

Thriving in the Present: Emily Infeld

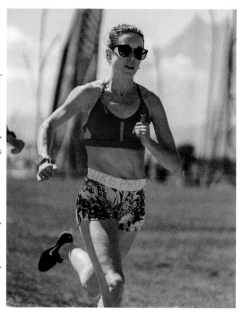

Courtesy of Emily Infeld. Photographer: Cortney White.

Olympian Emily Infeld has a lengthy list of running accomplishments to her name—a bronze medal in the 10,000 meters at the 2015 World Championships, an 11th-place finish in the 10,000 meters at the 2016 Games in Rio, and an NCAA 3,000-meter indoor championship in 2012.

She's also dealt with what she calls "a whole slew of injuries," including two sacral fractures, two hip stress fractures, a tibial stress fracture, and tendinitis in both her feet and ankles. But it's the hip surgery she had in 2019 that's had the biggest impact on her career, she says.

Emily had symptoms for about a year, but experts first recommended conservative therapies. Finally, she lost range of motion and struggled to pick up her left leg. Imaging finally revealed the culprit—a tear in her labrum, the cartilage surrounding the hip joint, as well as bone abnormalities. "I was told surgery of this extent is very hard to come back from and be competitive at an elite level," she says.

Though she felt frustrated and upset, she was also determined. To recover post-op, she focused on small goals—being able to walk without crutches, getting in the pool for the first time, and adding in more cross-training. She talked with other athletes who'd been through similar procedures and went on to compete successfully.

With that dose of optimism and the support of her medical team, she stayed diligent and made progress. She began her comeback in 2019—seven months after surgery, she placed fourth overall and first American at the Beach to Beacon 10K—and by early 2020, she began to string together more consistent performances, including a personal-best 14:56:33 in the 5,000 meters.

Now, she focuses on giving herself rest before she feels like she needs it. She swims regularly and every day does both prehab and rehab exercises. As she's posted on Instagram, "No body is perfectly symmetrical and my asymmetries have led to a lot of overuse injuries. Being aware of my specific asymmetries helps me target certain muscles with my strengthening and prehab routine."

She recommends finding therapists you trust, following your instincts, and focusing on progressing from where you are right now—not where you were before an injury or setback. "You know more than anyone how you're feeling; don't let anyone convince you to push through if you think you need to rest," she says. "And try as best as you can to not compare yourself to others or to yourself at peak form. You can only look at yourself at this current moment."

FROM BARRIER TO BREAKTHROUGH

Maybe you're 100 percent healthy now and looking to stay that way. Or you might be dealing with a minor—or not-so-minor—setback. Regardless, you can always set small goals to make progress, with an eye on the bigger picture.

Barrier

I'm not injured now, but I want to stay healthy.

Breakthrough Goals

Choose one or more.

I will do the following:

- If I'm falling short on rest or sleep, nutrition, cross-training, or mindset work, I'll go to the relevant chapter and choose a breakthrough goal to improve it
- Do full-body mobility two to three times per week
- Take 10 to 15 minutes in the next week to write out my injury history
- Consider my other risk factors and if I identify one, choose one way to counteract it

Barrier

There's something bothering me, but I don't think it's serious enough to stop running.

Breakthrough Goals

Choose one or more.

I will do the following:

- Take notes about how I feel after every run and mobility session for the next week so I can tell whether and when it gets better or worse
- Choose the mobility routine based on what's bothering me and do it two or three times per week
- Try a home treatment method to relieve pain and promote healing
- Go to see a health care provider I trust—or if I don't already have one, research someone who might be able to pinpoint the problem and advise me on what to do next

Barrier

Help! I'm injured right now and don't know how I'll still achieve my goals.

Breakthrough Goals

Choose one or more.

I will do the following:

- Allow myself ample time—for instance, 24 to 48 hours—to feel disappointed and wallow
- Consult a sports medicine professional for a diagnosis and treatment plan or if I'm already in treatment, write out my plan on the calendar the same way I would a training plan
- Revisit my goals and timelines so I have a new, realistic idea of when I'll make my breakthrough

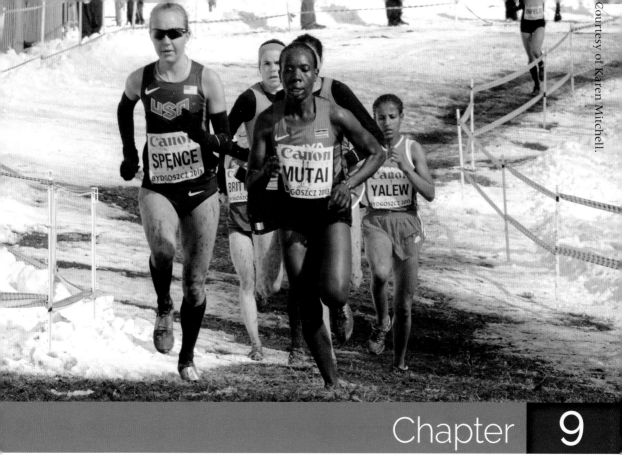

Chapter **9**

Exercise Your Brain

" Athletes must train harder, but they must also train smarter. Having a plan to improve your mental game is the key to " realizing one's true potential.

Dr. Candice Zientek, former sport psychology professor at Shippensburg University

" I always tell people when I speak, the fear doesn't leave. I was scared a lot of the time along my journey. But I got one of my mantras from something my pastor once said: 'Do it afraid.' You do it afraid if you have to, but you still do it, and then when you do it, each step just keeps getting revealed. "

Mechelle Lewis Freeman, 2008 Olympian in the 4×100 relay

Do you ever get nervous or anxious before a big race, lose your focus in the middle of a hard workout, or question whether you have what it takes to achieve your goals? I know I do.

But I *also* know there's a secret weapon allowing you to succeed despite those tough moments. You can call it mindset, mental skills work, or sport psychology; whatever name you use, putting conscious effort into training your brain pays off big-time.

With deliberate practice, you can build confidence, control your anxiety, and run your best. And even more importantly, you can have fun along the way.

A WINNING MINDSET

Heading into the 2013 World Cross Country Championships in Poland, I had every reason to feel nervous. I was joining a top-notch American team with Olympians, such as Deena Kastor and Kim Conley, and racing against runners from all over the world. We flew there just a few days before the race, which didn't give us a lot of time to adjust to a six-hour time difference. The day before, it had snowed heavily, and when we got up on race morning, there were six more inches on the ground. Oh, and did I mention that the course basically went up and down a ski slope?

All this could have easily thrown me off my game. I could have stressed out about jet lag, gotten intimidated by the competition, or freaked out about losing a shoe in the muddy moguls scattered around the course. Instead, I planned ahead, prepared the best I could for potential obstacles, and calmly coped with any unexpected challenges as they arose.

On race morning, I attached my spikes to my feet with duct tape, completed my warm-up, and lined up in the corral 45 minutes early as instructed. As I bounced around to stay warm, I took a few deep breaths and focused on myself and running the best I could that day. As a result, I had one of the best races of my life, placing first American and 13th overall.

It wasn't always this way for me. In the past, I'd had a lot more prerace anxiety. If things didn't go exactly as planned—if I couldn't eat waffles on race morning or do seven strides exactly 23 minutes before the starting gun—negative thoughts would creep in. *I'm way off my routine, out of my comfort zone. How am I going to be able to perform well?* I thought I needed a perfect setup to run my best.

This shift to flexibility and confidence didn't happen overnight. It was the result of years of intentional, focused work on mindset.

FROM DOUBT TO CONFIDENCE

My mindset work started the first semester of my sophomore year in college at Shippensburg University. That's when I walked into Dr. Candice Zientek's sport psychology class, one of the first electives for my coaching minor. She talked about flow—a seemingly effortless state of performance top athletes reach—and the importance of outcome and process goals. I was captivated, instantly recognizing how powerful these ideas could be for my performance.

I sat in the front row, hanging on to Dr. Zientek's every word. Before long, I appeared at her office door to ask more about how I could apply these techniques to my own training and racing. Unless I was traveling to a race, we started meeting for an hour every Friday.

Over lunch, we'd discuss how to create mental pictures of success, use mantras to reinforce them, and stay focused when it counts. Not only did I get an "A" in the class, I began laying the foundation for a successful running career.

Some people think mental toughness or positive thinking is something that comes naturally—or doesn't. While some athletes do seem to have an easier time enduring pain or controlling their emotions than others, anyone can work on mindset. Nearly all the world's best athletes dedicate time and intention to honing their mental game.

I find it helpful to think of mental skills just like physical ones. In the same way you practice, say, running uphill or sprinting to the finish, you can rehearse using imagery and mantras or reframing negative thoughts. Over time, you'll build a mental toolbox you can reach into on race day. The goal is to load it up so you'll find just the right strategy for any situation.

Of course, I still have negative thoughts and moments of self-doubt. Many of them cropped up after coming back from pregnancy and injury, and they even reappear when I race again after a scheduled break in training.

At the beginning of a season or a training cycle, it's harder for me to focus my thoughts. I have to be a lot more conscious about planning my mental strategies. Most runners, even the pros, experience this. That's why we call the first race of the season a rust buster. It's not just that you're physically readjusting to competition—you also have to remind your brain how to push hard.

But as I repeat and fine-tune these skills in training, they gradually become more natural. By the time I get to a goal race, they start to feel more like second nature. It's far easier to flow.

That day in Poland taught me that beyond a doubt, I could rise to the occasion if things went wrong and keep going when the going got tough. When low moments occur, I can overcome them. I've built a whole set of mental skills and practices through the years, techniques I continue to fine-tune and strengthen.

GETTING SOME HELP

Those weekly appointments with Dr. Zientek in college set me on the path toward a healthy, successful running career. And long after we'd shared our last brown-bag lunch, she continued to serve as a valuable source of support as well as being a friend. (I even invited her to my wedding!)

I highly recommend talking through the mental side of running with a sport psychologist or certified mental performance consultant if you have access to one. You can find a list of professionals certified to work with athletes through the Association for Applied Sport Psychology at www.appliedsportpsych.org. Coaches and trusted training partners can also serve as sounding boards for some of these issues.

And while we're talking about using mental training to improve performance, it's also incredibly important to talk about mental health in general. While running does ease stress and release lots of feel-good brain chemicals, runners aren't immune to conditions such as burnout, anxiety, and depression. In fact, as noted in a 2019 review of 52 studies published in the *British Journal of Sports Medicine* (Castaldelli-Maia et al. 2019), as runners, our type-A, goal-oriented personalities can leave us more prone to these problems as well as less likely to get help for them.

If feelings of sadness, anxiety, or being overwhelmed are starting to interfere with your running or your life, there is zero shame in getting help from a therapist, psychologist, psychiatrist, or other mental health professional. In fact, it's probably the best thing you can do for yourself and your running. And if you're thinking of hurting yourself or aren't sure where to turn in a crisis, you can call the National Suicide Prevention Hotline at (800) 273-8255 or text "HOME" to 741741 to connect with a crisis counselor.

The coolest thing about mindset training is that it can reach far beyond your running. Once you learn it, you can apply it anywhere in life. The very same techniques that help you crush a hard workout or cross the finish line feeling joyful can apply to challenges you face as a mom, a partner, a friend, or a coworker or overall as a human.

BALANCING OUT STRESS

As we've touched on in the chapters about recovery (chapter 3), nutrition (chapter 4), and pregnancy (chapter 6), you have only so much energy to complete all the tasks in your life, and on page 29, we even drew a stress pie. Once you realize you have more than a pie's worth of stuff going on, there are three ways to shift the balance.

Subtract Stressors

Can you ask for help with childcare or hand off a project at work? Anytime you can eliminate a source of pressure, you lighten your load. This could be a small tweak or a huge adjustment, for instance, changing jobs or moving to be closer to family.

Add Stress Relievers

These are positive steps you can take to offset the sources of stress in your life—everything from prioritizing sleep to watching a funny movie to investing time in your relationships. As a case in point, Dillon and I met in college, but he graduated before me and took a job that required him to travel from Sunday to Thursday. We started planning weekly date nights on Thursdays, when we'd watch *The Office* and get ice cream. (Honestly, it's still one of our favorite things to do as a couple!) Knowing I had that to look forward to made the time apart easier to manage.

Adjust Your Goals

For better or worse, some phases of our lives involve more pressure, and there's nothing we can do to change that. In those cases, the thing we can control is our expectations. For instance, maybe you can't go for a personal-best marathon and a promotion at the same time. In cases like this, there's no shame in adjusting your goal to something that will make you feel motivated, not defeated. Think back to my story about the Houston Marathon in 2020. I knew when I lined up in Houston that I couldn't run my fastest time but that I also had a goal—qualifying for the Olympic Trials—and achieving it wouldn't be any less satisfying than any of my other peak performances.

LETTING GO OF COMPARISON

Whether you come across other runners on the training path or you're eyeing your competition at the starting line of a race, it's human nature to wonder how you stack up. Social media makes this even harder to escape (more on that in a minute).

It's also incredibly common to compare your current self to your past self. If you're coming back from an injury or pregnancy, you might worry that you won't be the runner you were before. As we age, we fear we'll lose our speed or strength.

This is normal and natural, but it can definitely break down your confidence. Recognizing the issue can go a long way to defusing it. See whether you can catch yourself going down this particular rabbit hole and stop before you wind up feeling defeated. Refer back to your training log often and look for signs of progress. This shifts your focus to how far you've come versus the distance between you and others.

ABOUT SOCIAL MEDIA

Instagram. Strava. Facebook. Twitter. At its best, social media inspires, informs, and connects runners all over the world. However, we all know it can also lead to unwelcome comparison, stress, and negativity. Plus, if you change your training based on what you see there, you could easily overdo it and get injured.

Here's how I deal with bad feelings from social media and how I recommend my athletes do too.

- *Catch.* The first part is about being aware of what's happening. Notice when you're scrolling social media and you have a bad feeling from thoughts such as *I'm not working hard enough, I'll never be that thin or fit,* or *I should be doing that workout instead of what's on my schedule.* Be especially wary of posts that make you question your body image or trigger unhealthy thoughts about food and fueling.

- *Context.* Once you notice these feelings about a particular post or account, put things into context. Remind yourself that on social media, people are showing you the highlight reel—what they want you to see. Comparing that to your real life, outtakes included, is bound to leave you feeling like you don't measure up. (One great way to test this is to scroll back through your own stories and feed and look at them as a follower would. Your life probably looks pretty great from this view!) When it comes to amazing workouts from other runners, it's tempting to try them yourself. However, even if you see a detailed breakdown of times and paces on Strava, you're still not getting the full picture. What are these athletes training for and does it match your goals? Are they running in similar conditions? How many recovery days will they need afterward?

- *Control.* Remember that you have the power to change the way you use social media. If there is a particular account that always drags you down or triggers you, you can click "unfollow." I remember doing this when I was coming back after pregnancy—running accounts featuring fitness models with super-flat abs were only making me feel bad about my own body. Think about timing too. I've learned that in the weeks before a big race, I am more susceptible to self-doubt and comparison. I'll post on social media, but I won't spend any time looking at it. You could try something similar or use apps or phone settings that limit your social media time or block certain phrases or topics. And when it comes to workouts, sometimes athletes I coach come to me inspired by others' sessions, and often, we can indeed take ideas from other sources and apply them to our own training. However, we might have to modify them to fit our particular context. (When I post my own workouts on social media, I use effort versus pace; that way, a runner at any level can easily adapt them.)

Another way to boost your confidence is to try something completely new and different—preferably something that sounds like fun. Maybe it's training for a mile instead of a marathon (or vice versa), running more on trails than roads, or even biking or running an obstacle course race. This can reduce pressure, build different skills, and bring joy back into your running—and your life.

BUILDING YOUR MENTAL SKILLS

By now, you're starting to grasp the importance of mindset training. Here are a few exercises you can use to get your mental reps in.

Off the Run

These techniques allow you to practice mental skills anytime, anywhere.

Write It Out

Even if you've never kept a journal or diary, putting some reflections on paper can prove surprisingly powerful. I handwrite my training log with notes about how I'm feeling and often take the time to journal separately.

You can dedicate a regular time to write—such as when you first get up in the morning or weekly on Sundays—or use journaling whenever you feel stuck or frustrated with an aspect of your training.

Here are a few prompts, inspired by my work with Dr. Zientek, to get you started.

- *Best and worst.* Think about your proudest performance and the one that disappointed you the most. Document as many details as you can about each one. When you're done, compare the two and consider what you can learn from them.
- *Close it out.* As soon as you can after a workout, write down some thoughts and feelings about how it went. Over time, you can start to see patterns.
- *Free form.* Commit to a set amount of time—say, 10 minutes—and simply write whatever comes to mind. I recommend doing it by hand rather than typing. You never know what you'll uncover! Often, there are things I don't consciously realize I'm thinking or worrying about until my pen starts moving across the page.

Be Where You Are

We'd all love it if our life would align perfectly with our running schedule. But try as we might—even, say, planning vacations around recovery weeks and pregnancies around race dates—sometimes we end up with a lot on our plate at any one time.

Take college, when I was balancing exams with racing, or 2017, when we moved to a new house the day after the U.S. 25K Championships. And of course, every day of motherhood provides ample opportunities to fret about Athens and Rome when I'm running.

Nearly everyone multitasks at some point, and there are plenty of days when I'm momming, coaching, and cooking food to fuel my next workout, all at the same time. But when I start to feel overwhelmed, like I can't handle it all, I come back to a technique called compartmentalizing. Instead of worrying about parenting or other parts of life when I'm running (or vice versa), I try to take things one race, one day, one hour at a time, staying 100 percent present in just what I'm doing at the moment.

To make this work in practice, you can do the following:

- *Book ahead.* Sit down with your calendar and plan out how you're going to accomplish everything that needs to get done. That includes both life stuff—say, work projects and PTA meetings—and your training and race preparation. Block it all into your schedule.
- *Switch modes.* When you're running, put yourself in athlete mode. All you have to do is what's on your training plan for the day—you don't have to stress out about that presentation at work or what you're making for dinner. When you're off the run—say, with your family—remember, that's where you belong. It can help to include a transition of tasks, such as a change of clothes, a few deep breaths, or another conscious reminder to yourself when you're heading from one role to the next.

- *Stay on task.* We're all going to have those moments when other concerns creep in. I remember a track workout when Dillon brought Athens along and gave him an iPad when he wasn't supposed to have screen time until later in the day. I pointed this out on my recovery lap but then remembered (with Dillon's help) that he was "on" for parenting right then and I needed to focus on my workout. You'll see that this strategy sometimes requires giving up some control and letting people do things in a way you wouldn't necessarily do. (This is another thing that's really hard for me, but I'm working on it!) In that way, it's also good practice for letting go of what you can't control on race day.

Take Control

The mental drill in table 9.1—Stop, Start, Continue— comes courtesy of Carrie Jackson (Cindy's coauthor on the book *Rebound: Train Your Brain to Bounce Back Stronger from Sports Injuries*) (Kuzma and Jackson Cheadle 2019). It appears in that book as a tool to help you navigate the psychological process of recovery, but this version can be used to reach any goal.

It works well at the start or end of a year or training cycle. You can also turn to it whenever you feel like things aren't quite working the way you'd hoped. To do it, ask yourself the three simple questions.

Call It a Win

Some victories are obvious—my top American finish in the 2016 Boston Marathon is one that will always be special to me. But you don't have to wait for those major milestones or even to cross a finish line at all to celebrate. Giving yourself a big cheer, gold star, or cowbell ring for everyday successes goes a long way in boosting confidence and

Table 9.1 Stop, Start, Continue

Questions	Examples	Your answers
What do I need to stop doing to reach my goals?	"I need to stop doing two hard days of running each week because I always get injured. I am going to stick with one." "I need to stop squeezing in an extra cross-training workout per week because it leaves me feeling stressed out and I'm not sure it helps my fitness anyway."	
What do I need to start doing to reach my goals?	"I need to start lifting weights two or three times per week. I know a strong body leads to better running." "I need to start going to bed earlier. Sleep is critical to recovery."	
What do I need to continue doing to reach my goals?	"I need to continue running first thing in the morning. I'm more likely to stick to my schedule, and I feel far better the rest of the day." "I need to continue keeping a training log so I have even more data to use in this chart next time."	

From N.S. Gracey and C. Kuzma, *Breakthrough Women's Running* (Champaign, IL: Human Kinetics, 2023).

keeping you moving in the right direction. After I had Athens, I reset my GPS watch so I was constantly setting new PRs—it felt far better to log my longest run as a mom or my fastest postpregnancy 5K than to continually compare myself to the athlete I was before.

Some other things I've celebrated include the following:

- Finishing my first big workout of a new season (I'm always the most nervous beforehand!)
- Getting out the door for a run when I didn't feel like it or on the flip side, resting when I felt a niggle to prevent an injury (see chapter 8, page 109)
- Finishing my first long run of a training plan feeling good
- Overcoming a setback, such as the calf issue that popped up when I was preparing for the New York City Marathon in 2016
- Finishing my longest long run ever (This is a fun one to use for your first marathon—once you get to the race, every step after mile 20 is a new personal-best distance. You can feel proud knowing that regardless of your time, you're doing something you've never done before.)
- What small victories or signs of progress can you celebrate?

Stay Positive

Imagine that you see two groups of runners and coaches at the track. Both groups of runners are struggling. The coach of one group yells at the runners, telling them how terrible they are and how they'll never achieve their goals. The coach of the other group shouts out positive, realistic, and encouraging feedback: "This is hard, but you're strong—keep going!"

Which group of runners do you think will run better? And which coach would you rather have?

To me, it's obvious—I want to run for and to be the kind of coach that lifts runners up rather than tearing them down.

Now think about your own inner dialogue. When you're running—or working, or parenting, or at any other time in your life—how often is your self-talk cruel and critical? How often do you use negative words about what you don't want instead of positive words focused on your goals? And what effect do you think that will have on your emotions and performance?

Often, we runners are harder on ourselves than we'd be on anyone else in our lives. But you can achieve so much more if you treat yourself with as much kindness and support as you would a friend, child, or training partner you wanted to see succeed. Research bears this out—one German study (Walter, Nikoleizig, and Alfermann 2019) showed that eight weeks of self-talk training reduced anxiety and boosted confidence and performance in young athletes and that even one week helped.

Here are a few ways to put this idea into practice:

- For a set period of time—a day, a few hours, or even just an hour—use a notebook or your phone to track how often you say mean things to yourself ("I'm so slow!" or "I'm not smart enough to do this") versus building yourself up ("I'm strong!" or "I can handle this"). If you're tilted toward the negative, see what you can do to shift the balance.
- If you tried one of the previous journaling exercises, take an entry and look through it for negative statements, then reframe them in a positive light. For example, if

you wrote "I'm always struggling on tempo runs," rewrite it to "On tempo runs, I want to learn how to keep pushing hard even when I'm uncomfortable."

- When you're setting goals, make sure you frame them positively. For instance, instead of saying "I don't want to fade at the finish," aim to say "stay strong until the end."

See It First

Visualization is another powerful tool athletes use to boost mental performance. This involves mentally picturing yourself running strong, overcoming obstacles, or crossing the finish line. These just-for-you movies give your brain a preview of what success will look like—one that primes your mind–muscle connection so you can actually make it happen.

My dad and I are both big believers, but we use visualization differently. He could sit in a chair, imagine himself running the Boston Marathon or another course, and actually get his heart rate up as if he were competing! In his mind, he could paint a clear picture of the race unfolding. If a negative thought arose or a situation didn't go the way he'd planned, he could rewind and work through the challenge so he'd be even better prepared when the day arrived.

Meanwhile, I've tried to practice visualization outside of running and found it makes me more nervous and anxious. I have to be moving. So I use my long runs to "see" myself on different sections of a racecourse. During my buildups to the Boston and New York City Marathons, I would run on the treadmill at least once a week and pull up footage of the course on YouTube. This way, I could practice things such as how I wanted to feel at each part of the course and the mantras I would use.

You can try different types of visualization during your training cycle to see what works best for you—maybe you pull up a video, search online to find a guided audio script (some marathons, sport psychology pros, or meditation apps offer them), or just lie quietly for 10 minutes and think through everything you'll want to see, hear, and experience that day to feel strong, powerful, and prepared. Repeat frequently until you have the chance to make it happen in real life.

On the Run

Try these methods in training, then use them on race day.

Make Your Own Mantra

Mantras are words or phrases that when repeated, improve your performance. They're short but pack a big punch—you can use them to fix your form, transform a negative thought into a positive one (we already learned why that's so important), or remind you of your deeper motivation.

Some mantras might ring true to you throughout your running journey. "Trust the process" is one I love so much that I worked with a jewelry company to have it stamped on a bracelet. Another one I come back to, time and again, is "You can do hard things."

Note that there's a reason I say *you* instead of *I* can do hard things. Studies (Hardy, Thomas, and Blanchfield 2019) show that athletes can push harder when they use second- instead of first-person self-talk—probably because your brain receives the message as it would encouragement from a coach or friend.

Other mantras can help during a specific race or even a section of a race. One of my runners divided an entire marathon into 5K segments; I often break mine into thirds. Following are some examples:

- In the New Orleans Rock 'n' Roll Half Marathon in 2017, I used ABCs.
  1. *Attitude*, or an eye-of-the-tiger approach to racing
  2. *Believe* in myself and my fitness
  3. *Commit* to pushing hard at the end for a strong finish
- During the Arizona Rock 'n' Roll Half Marathon in 2017, I used Fs.
  1. *Find* my rhythm in the first few miles
  2. *Fight fatigue* in the middle
  3. *Finish* strong
  4. *Focus* when doubts creep in

There are many ways to use mantras. You can say them at every water break or every mile; write them on your hand or your singlet; or get a physical reminder, such as a bracelet or a necklace, to represent them. You might even work them into your breathing pattern. You can use my mantras or other runners' for inspiration, or check out your journal or running log for meaningful words, phrases, and cues. Make them personal. Even if your mantras don't make sense to anyone else, if they speak to *you*, they're good ones.

Break It Down

A long run or a tough workout can feel overwhelmingly challenging at the beginning. You can make it easier and a lot more fun by dividing it into smaller, more manageable chunks. Here are some examples:

- A 15-mile-long run becomes three, five-mile chunks
- A five-mile tempo run becomes one mile plus two miles plus two miles
- Repeats of 12 by 400 meters become three sets of four

Then make each segment a little different by using the following:

- *Mini goals.* For instance, on the five-mile tempo run, think of the first mile as a time to feel out your pace; the middle two, to focus; and the final two, to push hard.
- *Hydration and nutrition.* Sip water or take a gel or chew every five miles of your long run.
- *Gear.* This works great for track workouts or runs you do on a looped course. Do something different after each segment. Sometimes, I pull my sunglasses down, take off my singlet, and run in only a sports bra or even change my shoes.
- *Mental cues.* Switch between mantras or focus on a different aspect of your form. You might think about your knee drive for the first part, your arm swing in the middle, and keeping your shoulders relaxed as you push toward the finish.

Power Moments

I'll never forget that World Cross Country Race in Poland. Often, when self-doubt creeps in, I think back to how I dominated the narrow, hilly, snowy course. You probably have had moments in your running and your life when you truly felt brave, strong, and powerful, like you could do anything. Writing them down can help you recall them and restore your confidence. Following are some writing prompts to try.

- My best race:
- My strongest training run:
- A time when I wanted to quit but didn't:

"Impossible Is Nothing": Mechelle Lewis Freeman

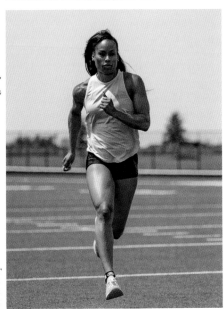

Courtesy of Mechelle Lewis Freeman. Photographer: Rebecca I. Flores.

Mechelle Lewis Freeman was a standout sprinter at the University of South Carolina. In 2002, she—and her twin sister—were on the team that brought the first NCAA Championship in any sport to the school. She wanted to train for the 2004 Olympics, but a hamstring injury held her back. Instead, she moved to New York City and took a job in advertising.

But the sport wasn't through with her yet. After watching her former teammates and competitors take to the track in the 2004 Games, she realized she could compete at the highest level—and still wanted to try.

Mechelle hadn't raced in four years. But she started training again, and her body responded. So she quit her job, got financial help from her mom, and moved to North Carolina to go all in on making the Olympics. "If you want to be the best, you have to put yourself in the right environment, around the people who are going to the same place you want to go. You control the controllables," she says.

One big element of this was managing her mindset—the books she read, music she listened to, thoughts she dwelled on. On her wall was a Muhammad Ali poster with the quote "Impossible is nothing." "Every day I would wake up, every day I would go to sleep, every day I was driving my car, I would repeat that mantra," she says. "I used to fold that poster up, take a little pin, and tack it up on my hotel walls wherever I was to keep that same consistent, grounded feeling."

The phrase—and her faith—carried her through. In 2007, she won a gold medal in the 100 meters at the 2007 North American, Central American and Caribbean Championships; silver in the 100 meters and 4×100 meter relays at the Pan American Games; and was on the gold medal–winning 4×100 meter relay team at the World Championships. And despite an injury that took her off the track for four months before the 2008 Olympic Trials, she made it to Beijing as a member of the 4×100 meter relay team.

Of course, her physical training helped her become one of the fastest women in the world. But without the mental and spiritual piece, she knows she wouldn't have endured through the injury or other tough moments, especially when others doubted her. "One day, I was in a cubicle in New York City. Two years later, I really was walking in the Olympic stadium, I really did run for Team USA," she says. "It took a huge mindset shift to make something like that happen."

FROM BARRIER TO BREAKTHROUGH

You've learned the importance of mindset work, and now it's time to set some process goals to put it into practice. Here are some ideas to get you started, based on the barriers you most want to work on.

Barrier

I fade during hard workouts or races.

Breakthrough Goals

Choose one or more.

I will do the following:

- Write down three potential mantras to try during my next workout
- Choose a workout, divide it into segments, and decide how to make each one different
- On a run in the next week, spend one mile envisioning myself running strong, smooth, and controlled or take 10 minutes outside of running to visualize a part of the racecourse

---

Barrier

I'm feeling stressed or have a lot on my plate right now.

Breakthrough Goals

Choose one or more.

I will do the following:

- Make a list of all the stressors in my life and come up with a way to subtract a stressor, add a stress reliever, or adjust a goal
- Make a list of one thing to stop, one thing to start, and one thing to continue
- Select a journal prompt, set a timer for 10 minutes, and put my thoughts on paper
- Set aside 10 minutes to block out on my calendar each day for the next week or if that's too much, even for one day, to practice focusing on one thing at a time during each designated time

---

Barrier

I'm lacking confidence.

Breakthrough Goals

Choose one or more.

I will do the following:

- Make a list of three or more power moments and keep them with me on a note-card or on my phone
- Choose one hour or one workout and commit to reframing every negative thought to a positive one
- Think back over my last week of training, identify three things I did well, and congratulate myself

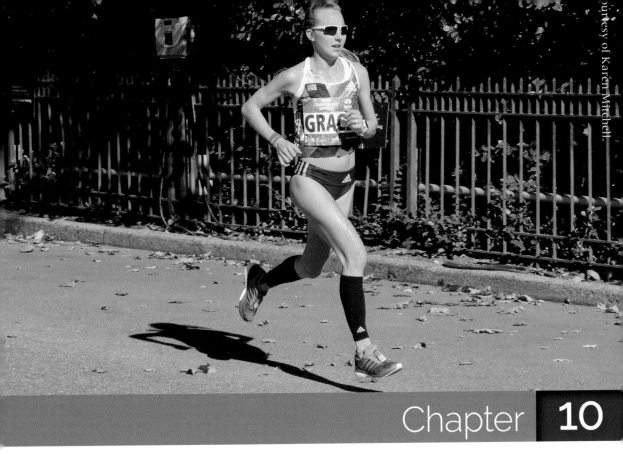

Breathe Better

" A simple deep breath while under pressure can completely reset your mindset, your running form and power, and lower your heart rate, which makes you feel much more confident. "

Amanda Nurse, Olympic Trials qualifying marathoner, mom of two, coach, and yoga instructor

We all inhale and exhale without thinking, but there's true power in bringing consciousness to the process while running. What starts with the simple step of noticing how air flows through your respiratory system can eventually evolve into a sophisticated system of counting breaths—one that when mastered, offers a huge advantage in races.

Learning to sync your breath to your steps takes time and practice but eventually allows you to regulate your effort in any conditions, stay calm and collected when you're pushing hard, and even gauge time and distance without a GPS watch or track markings. In some ways, I feel like this is one of my biggest secrets to success, but it's one I'm always happy to share with other athletes, whether it's runners I'm coaching one-on-one or those of you who've picked up this book.

A PATTERN OF POWER

It's hard to feel truly alone in a crowded city like New York. But during the 2016 New York City Marathon, I wound up running solo many of the miles, including the long, torturous climbs of the Queensboro Bridge, at mile 15.

When you make the turn off the bridge onto First Avenue, there's a long, straight shot ahead to the Bronx. With that clear view, I squinted, and maybe a quarter mile or so ahead of me, I could see the tiny speck of Sara Hall. Otherwise, no one.

Instead of feeling sorry for myself or freaking out about the distance between us, I turned my attention back to my breathing. In and out, over and over, I counted. My legs turned over quickly, my mind stayed focused, and I knew without a glance at my watch I was running the right pace.

In my head, I pictured myself right alongside Sara—matching her stride for stride, breath for breath. I could see us working together, with smooth and controlled form. Before I knew it, I'd caught—and passed—her. And even though I wound up hitting a rough patch in the last 5K, I repeatedly counted my breaths up to 100, over and over, to keep my head in the race. I wound up running a personal-best 2:34:55 (and finishing over a minute ahead of Sara, which was no small feat because she's an incredible athlete).

Even though breathing is essential for life and we do it every day, most runners struggle to get it right when they first start out, gasping for air before they learn how to pace themselves over a given distance. But after those initial hurdles, even many high-level runners don't spend a ton of time thinking about it and haven't unlocked all of its tremendous power.

Since way back in high school, when I wasn't allowed to use my watch at most meets, I've learned to use my breath to do the following:

- Calm down an anxious mind before a race
- Determine my optimal pace during a race and stay on pace, even when my GPS watch goes wonky or I miss a mile marker
- Relieve the side stitches I've struggled with for decades
- Adjust my effort between altitude and sea level
- Measure out an entire interval workout when I don't have access to a track
- Know without checking an app that air pollution levels are high and determine how much I can safely tolerate
- Sleep better at night
- Realize that I'm pregnant even before taking a test!

Doing some of these things involves techniques that are quite high level and complex, including breathing in specific patterns. Unless runners have experience in a sport or a practice that's more focused on the breath—for instance, swimming, yoga, Pilates, or even shooting or biathlon—using the breath to do these things doesn't always come easily. I might share these techniques with the athletes I coach only when they ask, and even then, they don't make sense to or work well for everyone.

But the athletes who are open to these ideas and begin experimenting with them find that they pay off in a more consistent pace, improved focus, and an ease of effort, all of which they value during hard workouts and even more on race day.

By mastering your breath—and especially a 2:2 breathing pattern (more on this in a minute)—you can run with more presence, reduce frustration caused by your expectations, and trust that you're performing optimally no matter what else is happening. Breath work brings a powerful sense of confidence to your running and racing, the assurance that you're doing exactly what you're supposed to do and getting the best out of yourself.

THE SCIENCE OF RESPIRATION

Why is the breath so important and powerful? Even though you can breathe without thinking, exerting some conscious control over the process can bring so many benefits.

Of course, everybody needs oxygen to survive. When you're pushing hard, your hamstrings, quads, and glutes thirst for even more of this life-giving gas. Oxygen is essential for the process of generating adenosine triphosphate, or ATP, the fuel that powers every muscular contraction. In some cases, your muscles' demand for oxygen can increase as much as 100-fold when you're training as opposed to when you're resting (Radak et al. 2013). The more smoothly and deeply you breathe, the greater the oxygen supply available to your whole body. The extra air translates into greater efficiency and power, keeping your stride smooth even when you fatigue.

Your breathing is also closely tied to your nervous system. Think about what happens when you're afraid someone's following you or you encounter a ferocious animal on a trail run. Your breathing quickens, your heart rate and blood pressure skyrocket, and you're primed to flee or fight back. That might help you sprint short distances to safety, but if the challenge you're facing is a marathon and not a mountain lion, you're going to hit the wall pretty quickly.

Assuming you're not facing life-threatening danger, breathing deeply and deliberately throws this process into reverse, releasing a neurotransmitter called acetylcholine, which activates your parasympathetic nervous system (Russo, Santarelli, and O'Rourke 2017). Your heart slows down, your muscles release excess tension, and even your blood vessels relax, all of which prove beneficial to covering longer distances. Even if you're in the middle of a challenging run, you can actively bring your body back into balance by inhaling deeply into the diaphragm, the major respiratory muscle.

As we touched on in chapter 9 on mental skills, these physiological effects go hand in hand with the psychological ones. When you're focused on your breath, it's far harder to fill your brain with negative thoughts or feel distracted by your watch or your competition. Your focus stays inward. Rather than expending energy on worrying about what's going on around you, you can channel every ounce of your effort into moving yourself forward.

WALK BEFORE YOU RUN

One reason I like breath work so much is that I can practice it on the run—I don't have to take any extra time out of my day to rehearse it. Not only is my schedule packed, but sometimes things like meditation and visualization off the run actually make me *more* nervous. All I do when I'm supposed to be relaxing is think about what else I could be doing with that time!

But it did take me a while to get comfortable with rhythmic breathing on the run. I always recommend that my runners begin their breathing exercises off the run first. Here's how to get started and then make progress.

Step 1: Try Belly Breathing

Start by lying supine with your feet on the floor and your knees bent. Put your hands on your stomach and take deep breaths, making sure your hands rise and fall—that means you're truly using your diaphragm and not just breathing into your chest. Inhale and exhale about 10 times. This is great to do right before a run.

Step 2: Take Your Breath Walking

Next, you'll start practicing that breath in a 2:2 pattern in slow motion. During a walk—for instance, on an easy stroll to the mailbox—breathe in for two steps, then out for two steps. Doing this feels weird at first, I'll admit, but it becomes easier with practice.

Step 3: Speed It Up

Once you're comfortable walking, try the 2:2 breathing pattern on an easy run. Start with just a minute or two at a time, counting two strides for an inhale, two strides for an exhale. Then give yourself a break before trying again. Work your way up to three minutes, then five, then a mile at a time. Eventually, you might notice you're breathing this way naturally on nearly every run—I know I do!

FIND YOUR RHYTHM

The 2:2 breathing pattern is by far the most important one. It's where I started, and the only one I used for a long time. As you become more comfortable with focusing on your breath, however, you might begin to experiment with different patterns for different paces.

At this point in my training, I've found that the following works for me:

- The 2:2 pattern works perfectly for workouts and shorter races, such as 5K and 10K efforts.
- For longer races, such as half and full marathons, or a regular training run, a 3:3 pattern (three strides for each inhale, three strides for each exhale) feels more comfortable.

THE STITCH FIX

One minute, you're cruising along in a workout or race, and the next, it feels like your entire side is on fire. I know the dreaded side stitches all too well—I've struggled with them since high school.

I know there's a hormonal link because they tend to feel worse the week following my period. I've also learned there's a lot you can do off the run to prevent side stitches, including hydrating; getting enough electrolytes; strengthening your core; and lengthening shortened muscles in your hip flexors with stretching, dry needling, or massage. Reducing anxiety or using stress-relief practices, such as the ones we touched on in chapter 9, also helps calm the nervous system and release muscle tension.

But when you're in the middle of a stitch, your breath can play a critical role in releasing it. My secret is to envision an "X" that spans from each hip bone to the ribs on the opposite side of my body, with the center right over my belly button. I breathe deeply, engaging my diaphragm, while focusing on that exact spot. I can do this even when I'm running fast—and it nearly always works.

- On an easy recovery run or in the recovery period between fast intervals, a 4:4 rhythm rapidly brings down my heart rate and keeps my pace controlled.

Some runners—including Amanda Nurse and four-time Olympic Marathon Trials qualifier Budd Coates (Coates and Kowalchik 2013)—use a staggered breathing pattern, such as 3:2. A longer inhale might help if you're struggling to overcome shallow breathing. With this pattern, you also alternate your foot strike as you breathe out, Nurse explains. During exhalation, with your diaphragm and core relaxed, your body's less stable. So by alternating which foot hits the ground at that point, you're more evenly distributing the impact on both sides of your body, which reduces your injury risk.

Personally, staggered breathing doesn't work with my natural rhythm; I find it distracting and confusing. Instead, I often distribute the impact by switching the foot I start with during each interval or each mile. That's where some experimentation by each runner comes into play—try it out during workouts and make notes in your training log so you can perfect the patterns that will work for you when race day arrives.

ADJUST YOUR EFFORT

Once you get a feel for your breath, you'll start to realize what a powerful tool it becomes to guide you through unfamiliar situations. By matching your steps to your inhalations, you can control your effort to ensure you aren't going out too fast or starting slower than you need to so you can account for the effects of the following.

Altitude

I live and train at 5,200 feet of elevation, where it's harder to breathe than at sea level. When I run on Magnolia Road—a popular route not far from me in Boulder—I ascend to 8,500 feet. Meanwhile, many of my races are far lower. Sure, complex altitude calculators exist, and they predict at least a 20- to 25-second difference between paces at those two levels. But I don't worry about targeting specific training paces for each location. Instead, I rely on my breath to help me slow down enough at high altitude and speed up sufficiently at sea level.

Hills

Even if you're a stellar climber, your pace just isn't going to be the same on the ascent as when you're coming down. Using your breathing to keep your effort level steady, however, can help you cover both sides of the swell as speedily as possible without burning yourself out.

Fatigue

The harder you train on your fast or long run days, the slower you'll go during every recovery run—and that's a good thing! There are a million other factors that also affect your body's ability to repair the damage from your last run, from your nutrition to how much sleep you got to the stress levels in the rest of your life.

Weather

You can't deny that temperature, humidity, wind, and precipitation have a real effect on your physiology. In general, running feels easiest at about 40 to 60 degrees Fahrenheit. But for the average runner, if the temperature is 20 degrees over or under that, the effort feels about 3 percent harder—so running an 8:30 pace seems more like you're pushing an 8:15 (El Helou et al. 2012). And anyone who ran the Boston Marathon in 2018 knows that finishing a race into the wind in the pouring rain isn't easy. But the exact degree to which these factors affect your physiology varies from runner to runner and can even feel different for the same runner from day to day, based on factors such as where you are in your menstrual cycle.

IN A FOG

In addition to everything else that happened in 2020 to 2022, wildfires burned through much of the United States, including in Boulder. On top of the devastation they caused for those in their paths, these blazes also made it hard to breathe for runners miles away from them.

Much like altitude or weather, air quality affects how hard running will feel. It also comes with other unwanted effects, such as headaches and a scratchy throat. While this is one more situation where tuning in to your breath can help you maintain an appropriate effort level, air quality affects your breathing not just that day but also in the future. So it's worth a slightly longer discussion. Here are a few more things to keep in mind regarding running in "bad air."

Track the AQI

The U.S. Environmental Protection Agency (EPA) tracks particles and other pollutants in the air using the Air Quality Index, or AQI. Many weather apps will note this information, or you can download a separate app, such as the EPA's AIRNow app. The higher the number, the greater the concern; while the scale goes from zero to 500, anything 151 or higher might pose a danger to the general public, whereas 100 to 150 is risky for people with asthma; older adults; or other compromised groups, such as children whose respiratory systems are still developing. However, you might notice that you're more sensitive and that, say, a level of 95 starts to slow down your runs. Make note of the numbers and how you're feeling in your training log, and pay attention to patterns.

Minimize Your Risk

On days when the AQI is high, there are steps you can take to reduce its effects. Run in the morning—especially effective in warm months—or on trails, away from other sources of pollution, such as traffic. You might swap days, cut a run short, or jump on the treadmill so you spend less time outside when the air quality is particularly poor. You can even run with a mask or an N95 filter on—something the pandemic has shown us isn't as impossible as we once thought.

Adjust Your Expectations

If you do run a hard workout or a race in poor air quality, don't judge yourself in comparison to efforts in cleaner air. Match your strides to your breath to gauge your pace, rather than focusing on your watch (sound familiar?). You might also allow yourself longer recovery periods between fast intervals.

Think Cumulatively

One long run or tempo effort in bad air might not be a big deal. But when you add up the effects of several days in a row, you risk longer-term consequences to your heart and lung health. If you are going to run outside in poor conditions, try your best to stay inside the rest of the day. Take at least some—or all if you prefer—of your runs onto the treadmill. During wildfires, I move my treadmill from the garage to the basement, where I could run in filtered air when I needed to.

Pregnancy

Because of all the other stresses on your body, when you're pregnant, your breathing will become more labored (pun intended). In fact, I actually knew I was pregnant before I took a test because my heart rate was elevated and I felt short of breath even during a 4:4 pattern! For as long as I was able to continue running, my breath helped me keep my effort easy.

The bottom line? By running with your breath, you're free from judging yourself against the pace you could've run in better conditions. Instead, all you have to do is maintain your rhythm, and you'll know you've gotten the best out of yourself on that day. It's a way of doing what's called "running by feel." This sounds somewhat emotional, which I think can be confusing, because with breath, it's actually a logical, tangible way to measure success.

A QUIET MIND

One more word here about the psychological piece. I mentioned how powerful breath work is in both calming your nervous system and slowing a racing mind. The great thing about practicing it on the run is the way it can pay off in other parts of your life too.

As I mentioned, I'm not big on meditating. But if I've had a particularly stressful day, taking 10 deep breaths at night relieves any excess anxiety and helps me fall asleep. Pairing breath and movement has also served me well in times when I couldn't run at all because of injury or pregnancy.

During those times, I cross-trained on the bike or the elliptical so I could still sync my breath to the movement of my legs. It felt familiar and reassuring, helping me hold on to a routine and a level of consistency I craved. I noticed that my anxiety levels dropped not only when I was exercising but also throughout the rest of the day.

When Athens was born, he and I would go on walks. I'd consciously engage my breath to keep me in tune with my body. I experienced a lot of postpartum anxiety, but once again, this practice of linking inhalation to movement grounded me. Step by step, breath by breath, I felt like I was returning to myself—and that even if my routine looked very different, I knew I'd be able to handle it.

UP FOR THE COUNT

Now, we're going to really get next level. Combining breath work with counting has, I believe, truly given me an edge in my racing career. It's what allows me to practice nearly perfect pacing without once looking at my watch—or even wearing one. With it, I've run effective track workouts without a track in sight.

It all started back in high school during those midweek meets where watches were forbidden. Often, these races weren't highly competitive. Instead of racing my guts out against high-level competitors—something I'd often do on the weekends—I'd use these races as workouts, doing intervals or Fartlek runs along the course.

But doing those races without a watch meant I needed some way to gauge both my efforts and how long to hold them. The 2:2 breathing pattern kept my pace steady. To measure time or distance, though, I needed to add a layer. That's when I started counting.

It's another lesson I learned from Poppa Spence, who'd used a similar technique in his racing days. Every two steps in and two steps out—one rep, if you will, of the 2:2 breathing pattern—counted as one. With practice, I learned that counting to 45 took me one minute. So when I had a Fartlek run that was one minute on, one minute off, I could count to 45 for each segment and know I was close.

From there, I started matching my count to a given distance. With my cadence, counting to 130 gets me to 800 meters, or a half mile. This came in handy once in 2012 when I was visiting Australia and didn't have a GPS watch. I had a workout full of 800-meter repeats, and the track was closed. So I hit a nearby grassy field and using just my breath to "measure" the distance, successfully completed the session. Now I may have been a few meters off, but I have confidence I accomplished what I needed to that day.

Even when I'm on a track or have a GPS watch to guide me, I still count. Since college, I've prided myself on my pacing—knowing just when to hold back and when to push through. I know this breathing–counting combo is what's enabled me to do this so effectively. So while it might sound intimidating or intense and definitely takes practice to execute, it might just help you push to your next breakthrough.

RACE LIKE THE WIND

Once you've tried these techniques in training, it's time to put them all together on race day. Here's how breathing factors into a typical performance for me.

Prerace

I definitely get prerace nerves, no matter how often I toe a line. But I've learned that this anxiety is actually a good thing—it means I'm excited and ready to go. Taking a few deep belly breaths before you line up can help you transform any stray butterflies into positive energy for your performance.

At the Start

As soon as the gun goes off, I start thinking about my breath. I instantly feel focused and engaged, and I don't lose any energy on distractions. This prevents me from getting sucked into the pace of the crowd and going out too fast—which I know would only make me suffer at the end.

On the Course

I count my way through the whole race, seeing how close I can get to measuring each mile with my breath. I'm usually within about 10 meters or so. Using my breath instead of staring at my watch means I'm tuned in to my body, adjusting my pace to match the conditions of the day. And it's especially helpful in big-city races, such as New York or Chicago, where GPS signals often disappear behind skyscrapers.

At Water Stops

These will obviously throw me off a little. But once I grab my fluids, I make sure to come back to my breathing rhythm before I drink or take my gel. That way, I'm not slowing down too much, and it's also far easier to eat and drink when I'm not hyperventilating!

Near the Finish

If I've kept my breathing steady for most of the race, I know that I'll have the energy I need to pick up the pace in the last stretch. In the last lap of a track race or the last three miles of a marathon, I finally start to push a bit harder, letting my breath get a little more strained. Once I see the line, I can finally let it all go and sprint as hard as I can to reach it.

CHECK YOUR CADENCE

There's yet another way that breathing can benefit you as a runner, and that's getting a handle on your cadence, or the number of steps you take per minute.

Legendary running coach and exercise physiologist Jack Daniels famously found that most elite athletes have an average cadence of 180 steps per minute during a race (Daniels 2021). Other studies have found that while that exact number might not be magical for everyone, a slower cadence increases what's called your ground contact time—the number of seconds your foot spends in contact with the earth on every stride (Schubert, Kempf, and Heiderscheit 2014). It's also linked to overstriding, which occurs when your foot lands too far in front of your center of gravity, decreasing the power in your stride. These factors can add up to an increased injury risk; fortunately, the evidence also suggests that increasing your cadence can mitigate it (Morgan and Vincent 2017).

If you're injured or injury prone, it's worth measuring your cadence. If it's slower than 180, increasing it could benefit you. Another red flag I see is when runners don't increase their cadence much if at all during fast intervals. Many GPS watches will measure this—if you take a look at your data and don't notice a bump when you're going faster, you might want to work on this.

Physical therapists typically recommend increasing your cadence by about 5 percent at a time. You can do it using a metronome app; picking a playlist of songs that are 5 to 10 beats per minute faster than you've been running (Spotify has lots of great ones); or using an app, such as Weav Music, which either adjusts the music's tempo to match your stride or allows you to pick a fixed tempo to aim for. Focusing carefully on your breathing as you aim to speed up your leg turnover can keep you calm and smooth as you go.

A Breath of Fresh Air: Amanda Nurse

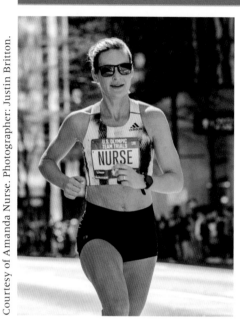

Courtesy of Amanda Nurse. Photographer: Justin Britton.

Amanda Nurse wasn't thinking about her running performance when she started practicing yoga more regularly in 2013. Mostly, she was looking to relieve stress from her job as a clinical social worker in a busy Boston hospital. "I found that when I went to an after-work vinyasa flow, I had the space to decompress from my day and, as a result, was in a much better mood too," she says.

Swiftly, the combination of breath work, meditation, and stretching she practiced on the mat translated onto the roads. That year, without changing much else about her training, Amanda slashed her marathon time from a 3:05 to a 2:54—then, with an even more focused yoga practice and more rigorous training, ran a personal-best 2:40 in 2015. The shift was so powerful that she became a yoga teacher in 2016 so she could pass this gift along to other athletes.

What she learned from her trainer, Laura Ahrens, solidified what she'd experienced. "The foundation of yoga is breathing—not the bendy yoga postures we generally think of," Amanda says. "The key that translates so well to running is that the practice of slowing down the breath has a soothing effect on your emotional state. The ability to focus on your breath, finding control in the breath, and deepening your breath allows you to stay present and focus on the current task at hand."

The techniques served Amanda particularly well during the 2018 Berlin Marathon. She was 10 months postpartum, stressed out, and sleep deprived. Just before the race, her husband learned that a work emergency would require them to fly home immediately afterward. Amanda barely made it to the corral in time, but once she was there, she took stock of her situation. "I remember telling myself at the start that I needed to focus on the here and now," she says. "That was all I had, and I still wanted to run the race I had trained so hard for."

She let her breath and her 3:2 pattern serve as her main focus. When the race got hard, she returned to it. She finished in 2:41—fast enough to earn her a spot in her second Olympic Marathon Trials. "To this day, this felt like a breakthrough race for me, one that I am most proud of for the perseverance and focus I exuded on a challenging day," she says.

As a coach and a yoga instructor with her own business, Wellness in Motion (WIM) Run Coaching, Amanda now guides her athletes toward the benefits of breath work. She'll have them start by adding 10 minutes of postrun yoga or a sleep meditation at night. When they struggle with short, shallow breaths during hard workouts—and panic sets in—she encourages them to do a quick body scan, bringing their focus back to a slow and steady inhalation. "Most often, figuring out how to control their breathing and relaxing their shoulders helps them navigate the challenging times and confidently get through their workouts and races," she says.

FROM BARRIER TO BREAKTHROUGH

Are you ready to tap into the incredible power of the breath? Whether you're an experienced yogi or have never given your diaphragm a second thought, here's how to float higher on air.

Barrier

I struggle with pacing myself properly or controlling my breath when I'm running fast.

Breakthrough Goals

Choose one or more.

I will do the following:

- Spend two minutes every day practicing belly breathing
- Add 5 to 10 minutes of postrun yoga to every training session
- Practice a 2:2 breathing rhythm on short walks first, then for one to two minutes at a time while running

---

Barrier

I don't know how to adjust my pacing for factors like how recovered my body is or what the weather's like. I'm always hard on myself for not hitting the specific numbers I'm supposed to in racing or workouts regardless of conditions.

Breakthrough Goals

Choose one or more.

I will do the following:

- After every training run, make a few notes about what the conditions were like and how easy or hard my run felt so I can match that to the numbers and notice patterns in how they affect me
- During each hard workout, experiment with different breathing patterns and make notes about which feels best
- See whether my cadence picks up on harder efforts and if not, take steps to increase it

---

Barrier

I already use my breath to guide my effort, and I'm ready to take it to the next level.

Breakthrough Goals

Choose one or more.

I will do the following:

- Experiment with different patterns for different paces and make notes about which feels best
- Experiment with counting and see whether I can start to measure out time and distance using only my breath
- Read about using breath during each part of a race and add in notes to my race plan about how I'll harness its power

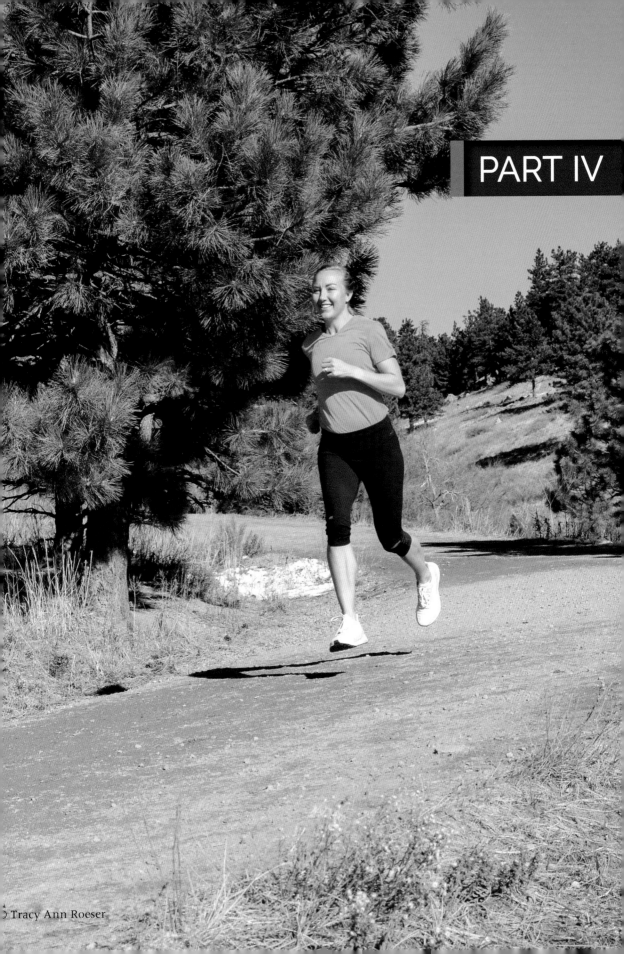

PART IV

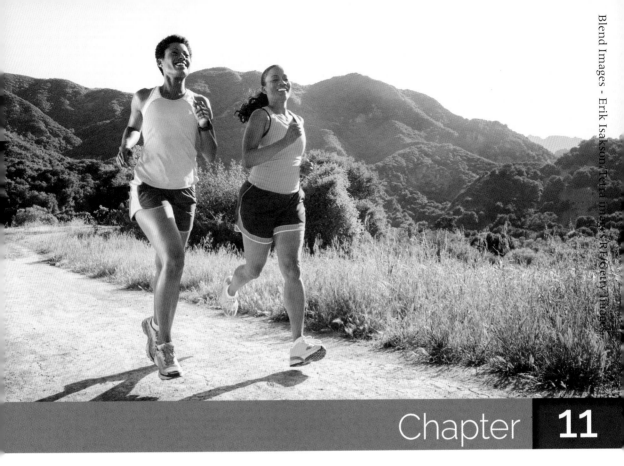

Chapter **11**

Let's Get Running!

The next few chapters outline training plans for a variety of distances—so many options for achieving your next breakthrough! This chapter provides you with a few basic details that apply to all the plans, for quick reference.

PHASE IN

Smart training begins where you are, then progresses you through a series of steps toward your goal. All my training plans include the following four phases, each with a slightly different focus.

Stability Segment

Many coaches refer to this phase as "base training." Here, you're establishing consistency and a routine that will serve you well through the weeks ahead. As you start to add in easy aerobic miles, you're improving your durability, the strength of your structures, and the efficiency of your running form so your body can handle harder workouts later on. I'll sprinkle in a few short strides—quick bursts of effort—to get you started on turning over your legs more quickly too.

Buildup Block

In this phase, you'll build on those strides to take your turnover to the next level. You won't be training much at your race pace just yet, but you'll start with some days that incorporate faster running, including negative-split runs, hills, and Fartleks. These runs improve your skills at shifting between different paces and efforts, which is critical to success in both workouts and races.

Performance Phase

This is when things start to get serious, with more structured and intense workouts and extended long runs that bring exponential gains in fitness. You'll also spend a lot more time at your goal pace, which trains your mind and body to find that rhythm. All this is meant to feel tough, but thanks to the first two phases, you're prepared to handle it. This is the best time during training to test your fitness in a race or two en route to your big goal. During this phase, it pays to be super dialed in, keeping your recovery runs very easy and focusing on your nutrition, sleep, mobility, and body work. Your peak week in mileage and intensity usually comes about three weeks before the race.

Taper Time

After you reach the peak in the final weeks before your goal race, you'll begin reducing your intensity and volume. You won't stop your workouts entirely—it's best to maintain a little tension as well as consistency in your schedule—but you also want to add in more recovery. The goal is to seal in all your previous efforts and show up at the starting line refreshed—mentally and physically primed to put in your best effort.

KNOW YOUR PURPOSE

In the plans in table 11.1, every run has a purpose, whether it's to increase your leg speed, train your body to burn fuel more efficiently, or recover and get ready for your next effort. Understanding what you're aiming for with each session and knowing exactly how to do it will help you make the most progress.

PRACTICE MAKES PERFECT

Training prepares you for race day in so many ways, but it's even better if you can get some practice in actual race efforts. Everyone has a different racing preference and style, but I typically advise athletes to race about once a month, starting about two months into a new training plan or season.

Racing at a range of distances will set you up for success in your goal race. For instance, if your A race is a full marathon, I'd do a half marathon or 10-mile race about four to eight weeks out, making sure to practice your fueling, pacing, and hydration. In other months, try 5Ks and 10Ks to hone your mindset and your finishing kick.

If your goal race is a half marathon, you might do one tune-up at that distance before your goal race and several 5Ks and 10Ks. And if your primary goal is a fast 5K or 10K, multiple test runs at your goal distance become a possibility.

Use each as a chance to not only capitalize on your fitness and notch a fast time but also to note what's working well for you—and where else you can focus and improve heading into your breakthrough race. Practice everything from your race-week routine to your mental skills to your fueling before and during the race.

You don't necessarily have to taper as much as you will for your goal race, but you will want to adjust your training a bit, both to prepare yourself to run well and to recover appropriately afterward. The training plans in this book don't include races because I wanted to leave you flexibility in scheduling based on the races available in your area. But you can adjust them or any other plan to accommodate. Here's how:

- The week before race week, consider cutting your long run back one to two miles or leave as is.
- Keep Monday's and Tuesday's training the same.
- Cut Wednesday back by a mile or two, or cross-train lighter than normal.
- Skip the workout the Thursday before and replace with a very light Fartlek or 20/40s (see page 155 for more about how to do these).
- Rest on Friday.
- Saturday, run an easy three to five miles with a few strides (such as the premeet session I typically recommend).
- Sunday, race.
- Monday and Tuesday, do easy recovery runs of four to eight miles.
- Wednesday and Thursday, resume regular training provided you feel recovered. However, if you have lingering soreness or fatigue, don't be afraid to cut back Thursday's workout a bit or even replace it with an easy run with 20/40s. If for instance, you raced a hard half marathon, you may need a little more time. And the risk of injury or setback here is greater than any minor bit of fitness you'd gain from the workout.

The biggest thing to keep in mind here is that you don't need to "make up" any "missed" mileage or workouts around the time of the race. Not only are you gaining valuable experience racing, but you're also improving your fitness out there on the course. Cramming in extra mileage won't get you any closer to your breakthrough and in fact, may set you back via overtraining or injury.

That said, understanding how to tweak your schedule also clarifies why racing a little too often can decrease your progress toward your bigger goals. The time away from training to prepare and recover is worth it a few times during the training cycle, but if you're racing every other week, you never have the chance to really get into a groove. And it's the combination of race experience plus week after week of solid training that will really offer you progress toward your goal.

Table 11.1 Types of Runs

Long runs	Here, you're logging time on your feet so your mitochondria—the tiny energy factories inside your cells—multiply and function more efficiently. It's a hard day but a different type of stress on the body than a fast workout. The extended time of movement trains your body to pull from the most sustainable energy stores. The mental component of the long run is also critical to your success—that's where you'll overcome barriers and boost confidence. On a few of your long runs, you'll run faster for a while or even gradually pick up the pace over the second half so you'll learn to stay strong when fatigued.
Tempo runs	Everyone has a slightly different definition, but I prescribe tempo runs at or near your predicted marathon effort. You'll see some labeled "steady state"—run these at the slow end of the tempo range, about 20 seconds slower than marathon effort. Meanwhile, the fast end of tempo range is no more than 20 seconds faster than marathon effort. These intense but not superfast runs train your body to use various fuel sources, making you more efficient at any pace and able to run stronger, longer. They're listed this way: Tempo at steady state 3 to 5 miles, 6 to 9 miles total. After a two-mile warm-up at an easy pace, you'll run 20 seconds slower than marathon effort for three to five miles, then cool down for one to two miles.
Alternations	This is a specific type of tempo run in which you shift between two paces, rather than locking into a single rhythm. For instance, you might alternate between your marathon pace and a steady-state pace. This type of workout helps you hone in on your pacing skills and teaches your body to recover a bit between harder miles. This skill comes in handy during many a race—say, if you slow down for fuel or water, then pick it up and find your race pace again.
Threshold workouts	Shorter and faster than tempo runs, these efforts fall right around half-marathon effort and teach your muscles to clear lactate and other by-products more quickly. A fun fact about lactate is that your body produces it when you break down carbohydrate for energy but it can also serve as a fuel source; these sessions are what train your body to do so more easily and efficiently. The higher your lactate threshold, as exercise physiologists describe it, the longer you'll be able to run hard.
Track workouts	Ideally, you'd do these on an oval in lane one, for precise measurements. You can also measure out a section of trail, road, or parking lot using apps such as MapMyRun, Strava, or AllTrails. Or you can even buy a measurement wheel and mark your segments with sidewalk chalk—that's what I did when the pandemic shut down the tracks in my area. Note that GPS watches may not be precise enough for short distances.
Repeats	This is the substance of what you'll typically do on the track and what comes to many runners' minds when they think of a "workout." Repeats mean short, faster segments; they're often 200 to 400 meters in length, at about your mile to 5K race pace, with substantial recovery. I find the time flies by! The purpose is to improve your anaerobic power and speed as well as making your form and stride more economical. In the plan, they're written this way: 8-12 by 400 m starting at 5K pace and working down on 400 m jog recovery. This means that after a two- to three-mile warm-up, you'll run 400 meters at your 5K pace, then jog 400 meters; repeat this 8 to 12 times, increasing your speed slightly each time. Finish with a one- to two-mile cool-down.
Intervals	These longer efforts, typically completed at your 5K to 10K pace, boost your $\dot{V}O_2$max and aerobic power. You can do them on the track if you like, but if you're racing on the roads like I do, aim to do them there. That way, you can practice moving fast and shifting directions on undulating terrain, instead of taking repetitive one-way turns on the track. When I have more than 10K of fast running on the schedule, I head to the roads. If these workouts feel challenging, you're doing them right—hitting this pace takes a lot of focus and makes the body work hard to recover.
Fartleks	This is a Swedish word meaning "speed play," and these runs can come in many forms. The type I prescribe involves running faster for a set period of time, followed by a timed recovery interval. You'll get in a harder effort without having to cover a set distance in a certain time, and they're perfect preparation for road racing because they'll teach you appropriate pacing. The shorter the Fartlek, the faster it should be run; aim for 90 percent effort throughout, where you are working hard but can recover in the amount of time given. Don't worry if you go out too fast and can't sustain the same pace the first time or even the first few times; this is a skill that takes time to learn. And remember, it's all about effort, so your pace may vary on hot days or hilly routes or during an intense training week. They're written this way: Fartlek with 8-12 by 30 sec hard on 90 sec easy, five to eight miles total. After a one- to two-mile warm-up, you'll run 30 seconds hard, then 90 seconds easy, then cool down until you reach five or eight miles, depending on whether you're taking the high- or low-mileage option.

Combo runs	True to the name, combo—or combination—runs begin with some miles at a tempo effort; a little rest; and then some shorter, faster running at the end. The goal here is to create some fatigue, then ask your body to push hard again—they're perfect for practicing a finishing kick, plus they make harder efforts more psychologically manageable by breaking them up into segments. In my marathon plans, you'll notice some workouts that start with a Fartlek, sneak in some tempo miles, then finish with a Fartlek—a fun effort that has you working on multiple systems and paces in a single session.
Hills	Heading up an incline is one of the best ways to enhance your power and strength without a lot of extra pounding. It takes a lot more force to run up a hill than to cover the same distance on flat ground—no wonder they make you so tired! You can do hills anytime after a proper warm-up. A 6 to 8 percent grade is ideal, but I know it's not always that easy to find. The rule of thumb is that the shorter the hill repeat, the steeper it can be. Ramps or parking garages can work in a pinch or a treadmill with the incline at 6 to 8 percent (though even Cindy, who lives in flat Chicago, can find hills within a 30-minute drive). From hill sprints of 15- to 20-second short bursts to longer repeats of 30 to 60 seconds, stay powerful and focused as you climb, pumping your arms and driving your knees up. You'll also see a hill surge run; for this one, find a hilly course and push hard on all the uphills and run easy on the downs and flats. Another run you will see that is particularly helpful for courses like Boston is a reverse hill surge run, where you will do the opposite of the previous workout and run the downhill segments hard.
Strides, including 20/40s	Like hills, these short bursts of speed break up the monotony of the daily run, improve the connection between your muscles and your mind, and keep your fast-twitch fibers primed for the next hard workout. I usually prescribe 20 seconds hard, about the effort at which you could run a mile race, followed by a 40-second easy jog. Take the opportunity to focus on your breathing, form, and overall technique while turning your legs over quickly. If they're part of a recovery run, you can do them anytime during the effort.
Negative-split run	Start out easy and slowly increase the pace and effort as you go. This is similar to the way I suggest you approach most races—so this is great preparation both physically and mentally.
Recovery run	This run keeps your body in a low-stress state. You'll recover from the training you've done and get ready for the next hard effort while still strengthening the aerobic system—critical for long-distance runners. Start off at the slower end of the pace range and gradually work into the faster end of it if it feels right—but if it doesn't, whether it's because of fatigue or external conditions, it's OK to keep it completely easy.
Rest	Days off are essential to allow your body to absorb the stress of training and bounce back stronger. On these days, instead of running or cross-training, prioritize recovery. Ensure you're getting enough sleep, fueling adequately, and engaging in stress-relief practices. Rest days are also good times to use assisted recovery tools like compression gear, massage, and heat or cold therapy (see page 30 for ideas).
Cross train	On these days, choose your cross-training method of choice, such as cycling, swimming, or the elliptical. See chapter 7 for more on the pros and cons of different modes. Keep the intensity easy to moderate so you're improving your cardiovascular fitness yet still allowing for active recovery.
Run/walk	You'll find these in the run-walk training plan on page 186. Alternating periods of running and walking will build up your endurance while allowing your body to adapt to impact. They'll look like this: 8×run 2 min/walk 1 min, which means to run for 2 minutes, walk for 1 minute, then repeat for a total of 24 minutes. Aim to keep your walking pace brisk and your running pace comfortable and controlled—these aren't sprints.

A BIT ABOUT PACE

We talk a lot about goal setting in chapter 1, on page 3. So you may well have a specific time goal in mind for your race, and that's fantastic! However, I always recommend athletes start training at their current fitness level, not at their goal pace. That's the best way to ensure you're properly stressing and adapting each element of your physiology. Start where you are, chip away at your fitness, and watch your breakthrough come to you.

Table 11.2   VDOT Values for Popular Race Distances

VDOT	Mile	5K	10K	Half marathon	Marathon
30	9:11	30:40	63:46	2:21:04	4:49:17
31	8:55	29:51	62:03	2:17:21	4:41:57
32	8:41	29:05	60:26	2:13:49	4:34:59
33	8:27	28:21	58:54	2:10:27	4:28:22
34	8:14	27:39	57:26	2:07:16	4:22:03
35	8:01	27:00	56:03	2:04:13	4:16:03
36	7:49	26:22	54:44	2:01:19	4:10:19
37	7:38	25:46	53:29	1:58:34	4:04:50
38	7:27	25:12	52:17	1:55:55	3:59:35
39	7:17	24:39	51:09	1:53:24	3:54:34
40	7:07	24:08	50:03	1:50:59	3:49:45
41	6:58	23:38	49:01	1:48:40	3:45:09
42	6:49	23:09	48:01	1:46:27	3:40:43
43	6:41	22:41	47:04	1:44:20	3:36:28
44	6:32	22:15	46:09	1:42:17	3:32:23
45	6:25	21:50	45:16	1:40:20	3:28:26
46	6:17	21:25	44:25	1:38:27	3:24:39
47	6:10	21:02	43:36	1:36:38	3:21:00
48	6:03	20:39	42:50	1:34:53	3:17:29
49	5:56	20:18	42:04	1:33:12	3:14:06
50	5:50	19:57	41:21	1:31:35	3:10:49
51	5:44	19:36	40:39	1:30:02	3:07:39
52	5:38	19:17	39:59	1:28:31	3:04:36
53	5:32	18:58	39:20	1:27:04	3:01:39
54	5:27	18:40	38:42	1:25:40	2:58:47
55	5:21	18:22	38:06	1:24:18	2:56:01
56	5:16	18:05	37:31	1:23:00	2:53:20
57	5:11	17:49	36:57	1:21:43	2:50:45
58	5:06	17:33	36:24	1:20:30	2:48:14
59	5:02	17:17	35:52	1:19:18	2:45:47
60	4:57	17:03	35:22	1:18:09	2:43:25
61	4:53	16:48	34:52	1:17:02	2:41:08
62	4:49	16:34	34:23	1:15:57	2:38:54
63	4:45	16:20	33:55	1:14:54	2:36:44
64	4:41	16:07	33:28	1:13:53	2:34:38
65	4:37	15:54	33:01	1:12:53	2:32:35

Table 11.3 Pace Chart Based on VDOT

VDOT	Mile	5K	10K	Half marathon	Marathon	Steady state	Recovery
30	1:08/200 m	2:27/400 m	2:33/400 m	10:45	11:20	11:40	13:30-12:00
31	1:06/200 m	2:23/400 m	2:29/400 m	10:30	11:00	11:20	13:15-11:45
32	1:04/200 m	2:19/400 m	2:25/400 m	10:10	10:45	11:05	13:00-11:30
33	1:03/200 m	2:16/400 m	2:21/400 m	9:55	10:25	10:45	12:45-11:15
34	1:01/200 m	2:12/400 m	2:18/400 m	9:40	10:10	10:30	12:30-11:00
35	1:00/200 m	2:09/400 m	2:14/400 m	9:30	9:55	10:15	12:15-10:45
36	58/200 m	2:06/400 m	2:11/400 m	9:15	9:40	10:00	12:00-10:30
37	57/200 m	2:04/400 m	2:08/400 m	9:00	9:30	9:50	11:45-10:15
38	55/200 m	2:01/400 m	2:05/400 m	8:50	9:15	9:35	11:30-10:00
39	54/200 m	1:58/400 m	2:02/400 m	8:40	9:00	9:20	11:15-9:45
40	53/200 m	1:55/400 m	2:00/400 m	8:25	8:50	9:10	11:00-9:30
41	52/200 m	1:54/400 m	1:58/400 m	8:15	8:40	9:00	10:45-9:15
42	51/200 m	1:51/400 m	1:55/400 m	8:05	8:30	8:50	10:30-9:00
43	50/200 m	1:49/400 m	1:53/400 m	7:55	8:20	8:40	10:20-8:50
44	49/200 m	1:46/400 m	1:50/400 m	7:50	8:10	8:30	10:10-8:40
45	48/200 m	1:44/400 m	1:49/400 m	7:40	8:00	8:20	10:05-8:35
46	47/200 m	1:42/400 m	1:46/400 m	7:30	7:50	8:10	10:00-8:30
47	46/200 m	1:41/400 m	1:44/400 m	7:20	7:40	8:00	9:55-8:25
48	45/200 m	1:39/400 m	1:43/400 m	7:15	7:30	7:50	9:50-8:20
49	44/200 m	1:37/400 m	1:41/400 m	7:05	7:25	7:45	9:45-8:15
50	43/200 m	1:36/400 m	1:39/400 m	7:00	7:20	7:40	9:40-8:10
51	42/200 m	1:34/400 m	1:37/400 m	6:50	7:15	7:35	9:35-8:05
52	42/200 m	1:32/400 m	1:36/400 m	6:45	7:10	7:30	9:30-8:00
53	41/200 m	1:31/400 m	1:34/400 m	6:40	7:00	7:20	9:25-7:55
54	40/200 m	1:29/400 m	1:33/400 m	6:30	6:50	7:10	9:20-7:50
55	40/200 m	1:28/400 m	1:31/400 m	6:25	6:45	7:05	9:15-7:45
56	39/200 m	1:27/400 m	1:30/400 m	6:20	6:40	7:00	9:10-7:40
57	38/200 m	1:25/400 m	1:28/400 m	6:15	6:30	6:50	9:00-7:30
58	38/200 m	1:24/400 m	1:27/400 m	6:05	6:25	6:45	8:55-7:25
59	37/200 m	1:23/400 m	1:26/400 m	6:00	6:20	6:40	8:50-7:20
60	37/200 m	1:22/400 m	1:25/400 m	5:55	6:15	6:35	8:45-7:15
61	36/200 m	1:20/400 m	1:24/400 m	5:50	6:10	6:30	8:40-7:10
62	36/200 m	1:19/400 m	1:22/400 m	5:45	6:05	6:25	8:35-7:05
63	35/200 m	1:18/400 m	1:21/400 m	5:40	6:00	6:20	8:30-7:00
64	35/200 m	1:17/400 m	1:20/400 m	5:35	5:55	6:15	8:25-6:55
65	34/200 m	1:16/400 m	1:19/400 m	5:30	5:50	6:10	8:20-6:50

Adapted from J. Daniels, *Daniels' Running Formula*, 4th ed. (Champaign, IL: Human Kinetics, 2022).

You'll see that I have paces listed for each run. It's critical to run your paces for workouts and recovery days. As you've just read, every run has a purpose—a system we are targeting on that day. You might find your easy runs feel very slow and maybe a bit boring, but they're critical to letting the hard work soak in.

For this plan, I prescribe paces based on VDOT, a system developed by the legendary exercise physiologist Jack Daniels (Daniels 2021). To find your VDOT (short for $\dot{V}O_2max$, which represents the amount of oxygen you consume during a minute of running), start with a recent race time. You can use any distance, but the closer you are to your goal distance, the better. If you haven't raced in a while or have never raced a 5K or 10K, you can do a time trial on your own where you aim to cover the distance as quickly as possible, or you can take your best guess as to how fast you can finish. Sometimes, I'll start my clients there. Look for that time in table 11.2 to locate your VDOT.

That VDOT will then guide you to the appropriate training paces. Table 11.3 lists the paces you should run for each type of session—from recovery runs to repeats—based on your VDOT. (If you've read Daniels' work before, you may notice these are a little different; I've fine-tuned them for women with big goals, based on my own coaching experience.)

Once you do a few workouts, you can adjust, especially if you're basing your paces on a time trial or estimate. If you're always struggling to hit paces and feeling defeated, you've probably overestimated your fitness and will be far more successful if you slow things down a bit. But if every workout feels easy, you can aim to train faster. I tell my athletes about the 80-10-10 rule: 80 percent of your runs should be status quo, 10 percent should be really tough, and 10 percent should be amazing. That ratio means that you're training at the right level and getting the most out of your hard work while not overreaching.

We talked about pacing and training by effort in chapter 10, on page 140. Once you start to get a feel for your breathing and effort level at each pace, you won't need to spend too much time staring at the numbers. But knowing what you're aiming for at first helps you train the appropriate physiological systems. Then as you get closer to race day, you can look back at this chart and the training paces you've successfully run to revisit your outcome goals and see whether you're on target.

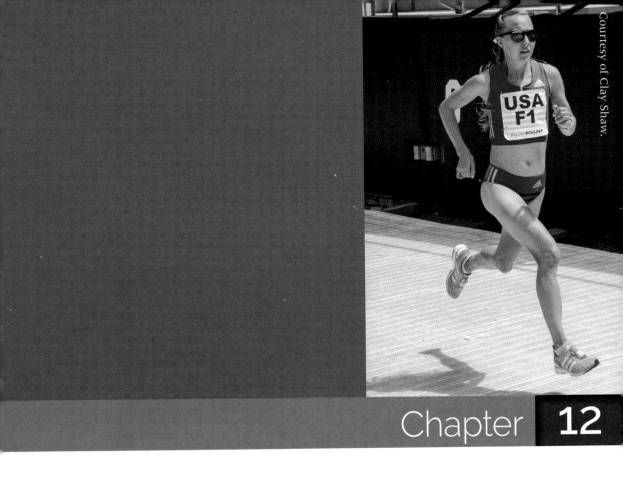

Chapter **12**

5K and 10K Training Plan

From Neely's Log

Breakthrough race: Stanford Invitational 5K, April 3, 2015

Time: 15:25, my personal best! This was four years in coming.

The field was stacked; among the runners were Gabe Grunewald, Marielle Hall, Emma Bates, and Alia Gray. The weather was nearly perfect and I was fit and ready. Prerace, I headed into the bathroom for one last nervous pee break. While washing my hands, I looked at my reflection in the mirror and whispered, "You got this." I ran strong, focused, and controlled, starting toward the back and passing people every mile. Each step brought new confidence, and although I never once looked at my watch, my splits told the story: 5:00, 4:58, and 4:50. I ran by feel, and I competed and rose to the occasion, placing fifth among top-level athletes.

GO THE DISTANCE

Though many runners hold half and full marathons on pedestals, the 5K and 10K also represent a significant challenge, offering an opportunity to test your speed and race at or near your $\dot{V}O_2$max. Training for them doesn't require quite as much mileage either, so you might find them easier to squeeze into a busy schedule. Plus, you won't need as long to recover after the race, leaving you ample opportunity to try again soon for your next breakthrough.

The plan in table 12.1 is 12 weeks long, with weekly mileage that ranges from 18 to 48 miles. Each run has a lower- and a higher-mileage option. Choose the best fit for you based on your current fitness as well as how much time you have to commit to your training.

Be honest with yourself about this—both ends of the spectrum will get you ready for race day. Some people have the time and training base to run more, but it's far better to run fewer miles consistently and without skipping the extras, such as strength, mobility, and adequate rest.

And about those extras, you'll see specific strength-training and mobility sessions built into the schedule. They're designed to build over time and to address the areas of the body that tend to need the most help at those points in the schedule. But of course, if you have other problem areas that you know need extra attention, feel free to swap them out or substitute (you'll find the routines and a lot more about strength training in chapter 7, on page 91, and find out all about mobility in chapter 8, on page 109).

RACE STRATEGY

Once you've put in the training, what's the best way to make sure you get the most out of yourself on race day? At either distance, I recommend a negative-split strategy—starting out controlled and patient, then gradually picking up speed. This approach not only keeps you from starting at a pace that's too fast for your body to physically maintain, but it also boosts your confidence, which is key to a successful outcome.

For the 5K

Think of the race as three parts, each about a mile long. For example, ideal splits would be 7:00, 6:58, and 6:55, with your hardest effort reserved for the last. Keep in mind that running at your $\dot{V}O_2$max is very challenging and if you cross the line into anaerobic energy production too early, you're unlikely to be able to hold on. I would much rather see an athlete save more than intended for the final mile than go too hard the first mile and tank—that's no fun for anyone, especially the athlete!

For the 10K

Stay focused and controlled through 5K, then gradually pick up the pace one mile at a time during the second half. This distance requires patience in those early miles; but trust me, it pays off in the end when you're pumping your arms and your legs respond with an extra gear in the final mile.

Table 12.1 5K and 10K Training Plan, 12-Week Schedule

Week	Monday	Tuesday	Wednesday	Thursday	Friday	Saturday	Sunday	Total mileage
1 Stability segment	**Recovery run** 3-6 miles	**Recovery run** 3-6 miles *Body weight routine*	**Cross-training** 30-45 min	**Recovery run** 3-6 miles *Resistance band routine*	**Recovery run** 3-6 miles Recovery *Mobility moves: lower leg and feet routine*	**Long run** 6-10 miles	**Rest day**	18-34
2 Stability segment	**Recovery run** 3-6 miles	**Recovery run with hill sprints** 4-7 miles with 5×15 sec hills *Body weight routine*	**Cross-training** 30-45 min	**Recovery run with strides** 4-7 miles with 5×20/40s *Resistance band routine*	**Recovery run** 3-6 miles *Mobility moves: lower leg and feet routine*	**Long run** 7-11 miles	**Rest day**	21-36
3 Stability segment	**Recovery run** 3-6 miles	**Recovery run with hill sprints** 4-7 miles with 5×15 sec hills *Body weight routine*	**Cross-training** 30-45 min	**Recovery run with strides** 4-7 miles with 5×20/40s *Resistance band routine*	**Recovery run** 3-6 miles *Mobility moves: lower leg and feet routine*	**Long run** 8-12 miles	**Rest day**	22-38
4 Buildup block	**Recovery run** 3-6 miles	**Fartlek** 8-12×30 sec hard on 90 sec easy Total: 5-8 miles *Body weight routine*	**Cross-training** 30-45 min	**Negative split run** 5-8 miles *Resistance band routine*	**Recovery run** 3-6 miles *Mobility moves: lower leg and feet routine*	**Long run** 8-12 miles	**Rest day**	24-40
5 Buildup block	**Recovery run** 3-6 miles	**Hills** 8-12×30 sec hills on 90 sec jog down Total: 5-8 miles *Body weight routine*	**Cross-training** 30-45 min	**Tempo run** 3-5 miles at steady state Total: 6-9 miles *Resistance band routine*	**Recovery run** 3-6 miles *Mobility moves: lower leg and feet routine*	**Long run** 6×30 sec hard on 90 sec easy in the second half Total: 9-13 miles	**Rest day**	26-42

(continued)

Table 12.1 5K and 10K Training Plan, 12-Week Schedule *(continued)*

Week	Monday	Tuesday	Wednesday	Thursday	Friday	Saturday	Sunday	Total mileage
6 Buildup block	**Recovery run** 3-6 miles	**Repeats** 8-12×200 m starting at 5K pace and working down to mile pace on 200 m jog recovery Total: 6-9 miles *Body weight routine*	**Cross-training** 30-45 min	**Negative split run** 6-9 miles *Resistance band routine*	**Recovery run** 3-6 miles *Mobility moves: lower leg and feet routine*	**Long run** 10-14 miles	**Rest day**	28-44
7 Buildup block	**Recovery run** 3-6 miles	**Fartlek** 8-12×1 min hard on 2 min easy Total: 6-9 miles *Dumbbell routine*	**Cross-training** 30-45 min	**Tempo run** 3-5 miles at marathon pace Total: 6-9 miles *Core routine*	**Recovery run** 3-6 miles *Mobility moves: full body mobility*	**Long run** 6×1 min hard on 2 min easy in the second half Total: 10-14 miles	**Rest day**	28-44
8 Performance phase	**Recovery run** 3-6 miles	**Repeats** 8-12×400 m at 5K pace on 400 m jog recovery Total: 7-10 miles *Dumbbell routine*	**Cross-training** 30-45 min	**Hills** Hill surge 6-9 miles *Core routine*	**Recovery run** 3-6 miles *Mobility moves: full body mobility*	**Long run** 11-15 miles	**Rest day**	30-46
9 Performance phase	**Recovery run** 3-6 miles	**Hills** 8-12×1 min hill repeats on 2 min jog down recovery Total: 7-10 miles *Dumbbell routine*	**Cross-training** 30-45 min	**Alternations** 4-6 miles running at marathon pace for 1 mile, then at steady state for 1 mile continually Total: 7-10 miles *Core routine*	**Recovery run** 3-6 miles *Mobility moves: full body mobility*	**Long run** 12-16 miles	**Rest day**	32-48
10 Performance phase	**Recovery run** 3-6 miles	**Intervals** 6-8×800 m starting at 10K and working down to 5K on 400 m jog Total: 7-10 miles *Dumbbell routine*	**Cross-training** 30-45 min	**Fartlek** 2×30 sec on 60 sec, 2×1 min on 90 sec, 2×2 min on 2 min, 2×1 min on 90 sec, 2×30 sec on 60 sec Total: 6-9 miles *Core routine*	**Recovery run** 3-6 miles *Mobility moves: full body mobility*	**Long run** Progression (start out easy for the first half, then progress the pace the second half as feels right to you) Total: 10-14 miles	**Rest day**	29-45

Week	Monday	Tuesday	Wednesday	Thursday	Friday	Saturday	Sunday	Total mileage
11 Taper time	**Recovery run** 3-6 miles	**Threshold workout** 3-5×1 mile repeats starting at half marathon pace and working down to 10K or 5K on 400 m jog Total: 6-9 miles *Dumbbell routine*	**Cross-training** 30-45 min	**Combo workout** 2-3 miles at marathon pace, 400 m jog, 4×400 m at 5K on 400 m jog Total: 7-9 miles *Core routine*	**Recovery run** 3-6 miles *Mobility moves: full body mobility*	**Long run** 8-11 miles	**Rest day**	27-41
12 Taper time	**Recovery run** 3-6 miles	**Fartlek** 2×1 min hard on 2 min easy, 4×30 sec hard on 90 sec easy Total: 5-7 miles *Dumbbell routine*	**Cross-training** 30-45 min	**Recovery run with strides** 4 miles with 5×20/40s *Core routine*	**Rest day** *Mobility moves: full body mobility*	**Premeet** 3 miles easy with strides	**Race day** 2-mile warm-up, 1-mile cool down	20-29

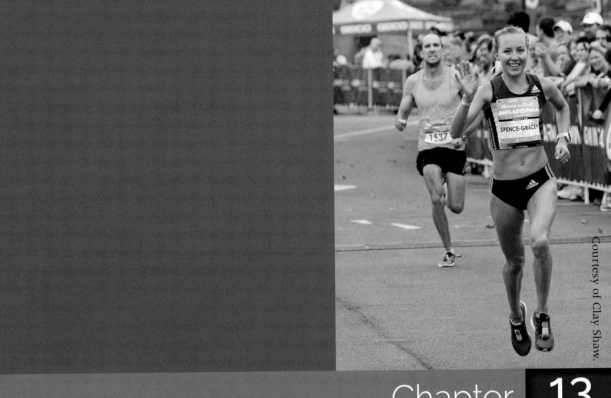

Chapter **13**

Half-Marathon Training Plan

From Neely's Log

Breakthrough race: Philly Rock 'n' Roll Half Marathon, October 31, 2015

Time: 69:59, second place

This was a year of beginnings: a new home in Colorado; running pro without a training group; a step up to longer distances; and even a new family member, our four-month-old Vizsla, Strider! It was a lot to balance—puppy training is no joke—but I loved my new life, and because of that, my running thrived. Early on, I'd set a goal to race a half marathon in under 71 minutes this season. But after a series of strong performances, I started to wonder if I could go even faster and run under 70 minutes. This particular race, my third try at the distance, didn't start off as smoothly as I'd hoped. The elite bus broke down, so we arrived late to the start. I missed doing my drills and strides. But I used the first three miles as a warm-up, cranked in the last few, and surprised even myself when I saw the clock at the finish. This made me the 11th American woman ever to break 70 minutes in the distance—an accomplishment no one can ever take away from me. And it gave me a huge boost of confidence for moving up to the marathon.

GO THE DISTANCE

It's true confession time—the half marathon is my absolute favorite distance. And I'm not alone. According to the annual State of Running report by RunRepeat, it's the second most popular, after the 5K (Andersen 2021).

An entire 13.1 miles sounds long and intimidating to some (including high school Neely, who loved the mile most). Completing this distance—and especially, racing it to your fullest potential—definitely represents a true accomplishment. However, the training doesn't quite consume your life the way marathon training does. Add this to the fact that it's much more common than the 10K, and you just might realize it's the perfect setting for a breakthrough.

This plan is 16 weeks long, with weekly mileage that ranges from 22 to 55 miles (see table 13.1). Each run has a lower- and a higher-mileage option. Ideally, you'd choose one end of the scale (or the middle) and stick with that distance through the whole training plan. To decide, take a look at your current mileage—you should start close to where you are now, rather than making a huge jump in just the first week—and determine how much time you have in your schedule to train.

Rest assured that all the options will get you ready for race day; even the lower-mileage option has a long run that takes you over the distance of the race itself. So if you're not sure, I recommend being more conservative. That way, you'll have plenty of time to incorporate the prescribed strength and mobility exercises. As you move up in distance, those routines—as well as adequate rest—are even more critical to staying healthy and performing well.

You'll find all the strength exercises in chapter 7, on page 94, and mobility moves in chapter 8, on page 114. I've added these components to the schedule in a progressive fashion and with an eye toward the muscles and joints that tend to tighten up with added mileage. However, feel free to swap out or substitute other routines that target your individual problem areas.

RACE STRATEGY

Patience and persistence are the name of the game with this distance. I recommend breaking the race into four segments.

1. *Miles one to three.* Ease in with a relaxed start, gradually working up to your goal pace by the third mile. Don't let the starting-line excitement carry you away—your goal pace may feel easy now, but you'll want to conserve adequate energy for the later miles.

2. *Miles three to seven.* Stay calm and relaxed at your goal pace. Keep your focus on your body and breathing. I find a 2:2 pattern works best.

3. *Miles 7 to 10.* These miles may feel the most grueling. Save your most meaningful mantra for this segment. Remind yourself of all the hard work you did to prepare. Soak up the energy of the crowd and the runners around you and visualize the finish line.

4. *Miles 10 to the finish.* The race is on! Kick it in to a strong finish with everything you've got.

To run your best at this distance, you'll need to take in fluids and fuel on the course. There's a lot more about nutrition in chapter 4, on page 37, but in brief, I recommend a gel about 5 to 10 minutes before the gun goes off, sipping water or electrolyte drinks at aid stations along the course (or carrying your own), and taking another gel at six miles. What's most important, though, is practicing during your long runs in training so you know what will work for you and your gut.

Table 13.1 Half-Marathon Training Plan, 16-Week Schedule

Week	Monday	Tuesday	Wednesday	Thursday	Friday	Saturday	Sunday	Total mileage
1 Stability segment	**Recovery run** 4-7 miles	**Recovery run** 4-7 miles *Core routine*	**Cross-training** 30-60 min	**Recovery run** 4-7 miles *Core routine*	**Recovery run** 3-6 miles *Mobility moves: tight hips*	**Long run** 7-10 miles	Rest day	22-37
2 Stability segment	**Recovery run** 4-7 miles	**Recovery run** 4-7 miles *Core routine*	**Cross-training** 30-60 min	**Recovery run** 4-7 miles *Core routine*	**Recovery run** 3-6 miles *Mobility moves: tight hips*	**Long run** 8-11 miles	Rest day	23-38
3 Stability segment	**Recovery run** 4-7 miles	**Recovery run with strides** 4-7 miles with 5×20/40s *Core routine*	**Cross-training** 30-60 min	**Recovery run with strides** 4-7 miles with 5×20/40s *Core routine*	**Recovery run** 3-6 miles *Mobility moves: tight hips*	**Long run** 8-11 miles	Rest day	23-38
4 Stability segment	**Recovery run** 4-7 miles	**Recovery run with strides** 5-8 miles with 5×20/40s *Core routine*	**Cross-training** 30-60 min	**Recovery run with strides** 5-8 miles with 5×20/40s *Core routine*	**Recovery run** 4-7 miles *Mobility moves: tight hips*	**Long run** 9-12 miles	Rest day	27-42
5 Stability segment	**Recovery run** 4-7 miles	**Recovery run with hill sprints** 5-8 miles with 5×15 sec hill sprints *Body weight routine*	**Cross-training** 30-60 min	**Recovery run with hill sprints** 5-8 miles with 5×15 sec hill sprints *Body weight routine*	**Recovery run** 4-7 miles *Mobility moves: lower legs and feet*	**Long run** 6×30 sec hard on 90 sec easy in the second half Total: 9-12 miles	Rest day	27-42
6 Stability segment	**Recovery run** 4-7 miles	**Recovery run with hill sprints** 6-9 miles with 5×15 sec hill sprints *Body weight routine*	**Cross-training** 30-60 min	**Recovery run with hill sprints** 6-9 miles with 5×15 sec hill sprints *Body weight routine*	**Recovery run** 4-7 miles *Mobility moves: lower legs and feet*	**Long run** 10-13 miles	Rest day	30-45

Week	Monday	Tuesday	Wednesday	Thursday	Friday	Saturday	Sunday	Total mileage
7 Buildup block	**Recovery run** 4-7 miles	**Fartlek** 2 sets of 4-8×30 sec hard on 90 sec easy with 3 min between sets Total: 6-9 miles *Body weight routine*	**Cross-training** 30-60 min	**Negative-split run** 6-9 miles *Body weight routine*	**Recovery run** 4-7 miles *Mobility moves: lower legs and feet*	**Long run** 6×1 min hard on 3 min easy in the second half Total: 10-13 miles	**Rest day**	30-45
8 Buildup block	**Recovery run** 5-8 miles	**Repeats** 2 sets of 6-8×200 m at 5K-1 mile pace on 200 m jog with 400 m jog between sets Total: 7-10 miles *Body weight routine*	**Cross-training** 30-60 min	**Hill surge run** 7-10 miles *Body weight routine*	**Recovery run** 4-7 miles *Mobility moves: lower legs and feet*	**Long run** 11-14 miles	**Rest day**	34-49
9 Buildup block	**Recovery run** 5-8 miles	**Hills** 2 sets of 4-8×30 sec hills on 90 sec easy jog down recovery with 3 min recovery between sets Total: 7-10 miles *Dumbbell routine*	**Cross-training** 30-60 min	**Fartlek** 4×2 min hard on 2 min easy, 4×1 min hard on 2 min easy, 4×30 sec hard on 90 sec easy Total: 7-10 miles *Dumbbell routine*	**Recovery run** 4-7 miles *Mobility moves: knee pain or stiffness*	**Long run** 4 miles easy, 3-5 miles alternating between marathon pace and steady state every mile (start and end with a marathon-pace mile), easy miles to finish out total volume Total: 11-14 miles	**Rest day**	34-49
10 Buildup block	**Recovery run with hill sprints** 6-9 miles with 5×15 sec hills	**Intervals** 3-4 sets of 4×400 m at half-marathon-10K pace on 100 m jog with 400 m jog between sets Total: 7-10 miles *Dumbbell routine*	**Cross-training** 30-60 min	**Negative-split run** 7-10 miles *Dumbbell routine*	**Recovery run** 4-7 miles *Mobility moves: knee pain or stiffness*	**Long run** 12-15 miles	**Rest day**	36-51

(continued)

Table 13.1 Half-Marathon Training Plan, 16-Week Schedule *(continued)*

Week	Monday	Tuesday	Wednesday	Thursday	Friday	Saturday	Sunday	Total mileage
11 Performance phase	**Recovery run with strides** 6-9 miles with 5×20/40s	**Hills** 4×1 min hill, 4×45 sec hill, 4×30 sec hill, all on easy jog down recovery Total: 7-10 miles *Dumbbell routine*	**Cross-training** 30-60 min	**Combo run** 3-5 miles at steady state, 400 m jog, 4×30 sec hard on 90 sec easy Total: 7-10 miles *Dumbbell routine*	**Recovery run** 5-8 miles *Mobility moves: knee pain or stiffness*	**Long run** 4 miles easy, 2-3×2 miles at marathon pace with 1 mile easy between, easy miles to finish out total run Total: 12-15 miles	**Rest day**	37-52
12 Performance phase	**Recovery run with hill sprints** 6-9 miles with 5×15 sec hill sprints	**Intervals** 2 sets of 3-4×800 m at half-marathon-10K on 200 m jog with 400 m jog between sets Total: 7-10 miles *Dumbbell routine*	**Cross-training** 30-60 min	**Tempo run** 4-6 miles at marathon pace Total: 8-11 miles *Dumbbell routine*	**Recovery run** 5-8 miles *Mobility moves: knee pain or stiffness*	**Long run** 13-16 miles	**Rest day**	39-54
13 Performance phase	**Recovery run with strides** 6-9 miles with 5×20/40s	**Fartlek** 3×3 min hard, 3×2 min hard, 3×1 min hard all on 2 min easy Total: 7-10 miles *Resistance band routine*	**Cross-training** 30-60 min	**Threshold workout** 4-6×1 mile at half-marathon pace on 400 jog recovery 8-10 miles *Resistance band routine*	**Recovery run** 5-8 miles *Mobility moves: full-body mobility*	**Long run** 14-17 miles	**Rest day**	40-55
14 Performance phase	**Recovery run** 6-9 miles	**Recovery run with strides** 7-10 miles with 8×20/40s *Resistance band routine*	**Cross-training** 30-60 min	**Threshold workout** 2-3×2 miles at half-marathon pace on 400 m jog Total: 8-11 miles *Resistance band routine*	**Recovery run** 5-8 miles *Mobility moves: full-body mobility*	**Long run** Progression (start out easy for the first half, then progress the pace the second half as feels right to you) Total: 10-13 miles	**Rest day**	36-51

Week	Monday	Tuesday	Wednesday	Thursday	Friday	Saturday	Sunday	Total mileage
15 Taper time	**Recovery run with hill sprints** 6-9 miles with 5×15 sec hill sprints	**Fartlek** 8-12×1 min hard on 2 min easy Total: 6-9 miles *Resistance band routine*	**Cross-training** 30-60 min	**Combo run** 1-2 sets of 1 mile at steady state on 1 min jog, 1 mile at marathon pace on 2 min jog, 1 mile at half-marathon pace on 3 min jog Total: 6-9 miles *Resistance band routine*	**Recovery run** 5-8 miles *Mobility moves: full-body mobility*	**Long run** 8-11 miles	**Rest day**	30-45
16 Taper time	**Recovery run** 4-7 miles	**Combo run** 2 miles at marathon pace, 2-4×400 m at half-marathon pace all on 400 m jog Total: 6-8 miles *Resistance band routine*	**Cross-training** 30-60 min	**Recovery run** 4-7 miles *Resistance band routine*	**Rest day** *Mobility moves: full-body mobility*	**Premeet** 3 miles easy with strides	**Half-marathon race** 13.1 miles (1- to 2-mile warm-up)	30-38

171

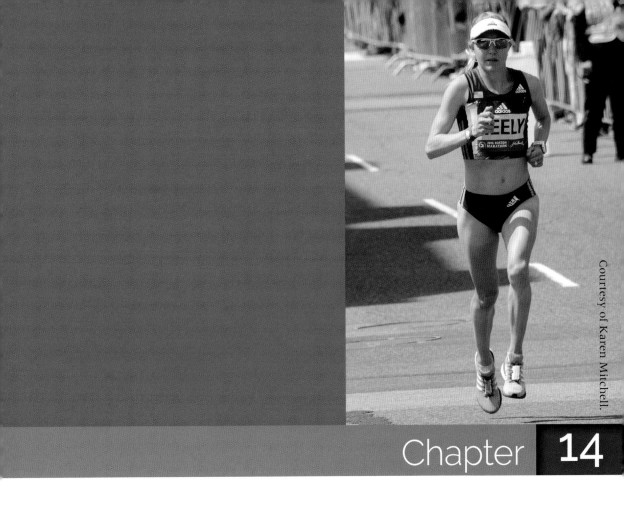

Chapter **14**

Marathon Training Plan

From Neely's Log

Breakthrough race New York City Marathon, November 6, 2016

Time: 2:34:55, eighth place and second American

Looking back on the past five months of focus, I am proud of my efforts. I had my highest-mileage week ever at 110, ran my longest training run ever of 22.5 miles, stayed healthy overall, and felt continual progression with each week. Most importantly, I enjoyed the process as I worked toward this marathon goal. The night before, not knowing how the race would play out, I felt a sense of satisfaction already knowing I prepared well, and I arrived at the starting line with a smile on my face. This race was a challenging one—I definitely hit the notorious wall in the last 5K. But I stayed strong and made it to the finish line in a personal-best time. There's no doubt in my mind now: I'm meant to be here, and I have what it takes to be a world-class marathoner.

GO THE DISTANCE

I probably don't have to tell you that there's something magical about the marathon distance. For many runners, going the full 26.2 represents the pinnacle of athletic achievement.

Maybe it's the storied history. Inspired by the journey of the Greek soldier Pheidippides in 490 BC, the first Olympic Marathon was held at the Athens Games in 1896. (And yes, that's exactly why we named our first child Athens.) Or it may be the unbelievable energy and excitement of the fans and crowds at World Marathon Majors, such as Boston, New York, and Chicago.

For women, the marathon holds the special distinction of being one of the final frontiers of running; we weren't allowed to compete in it until 1984, nearly 100 years after its inaugural running. When American Joan Benoit Samuelson entered the Olympic Stadium in Los Angeles waving her white hat, en route to winning the first-ever gold in the event, she laid the groundwork for legions of us to have breakthroughs after her.

While we've long since proven female bodies are strong enough to withstand a marathon effort, it's true that getting ready for 26.2 miles requires respect, dedication, and a *lot* of time and energy. This training plan is 22 weeks long—that's more than five months of dedicated, focused preparation (see table 14.1).

As we discussed in chapter 2, marathon training is unique in that for the vast majority of athletes, the full distance of the race is too taxing to do in training. A variety of other types of workouts—long runs, tempo and steady-state runs, and faster repeats and intervals—combine to create the type of fatigue that prepares your body to hold race pace for such an extended distance. Of course, all that must be balanced with adequate rest and recovery to reap the benefits.

It's a tricky balance, one that requires both a well-designed plan, such as this one, and having some flexibility to listen to your body. Some days, you may surprise yourself and go faster or longer than what you expected. On the flip side, some days feel tougher. Don't be afraid to run slower or cut a workout short if you're sore, excessively fatigued, or otherwise seem underrecovered. It's important to defer to your body's signals in any type of training, but when you're preparing for the marathon, it's even more crucial than usual.

And marathon training is when dialing in all the other details—from sleep to hydration to nutrition and mobility work—truly becomes critical. I always believe well-rounded athletes are the happiest and healthiest, but training to run your best marathon more often requires trade-offs and small sacrifices. For instance, you might choose to stay in Friday night when your long run is Saturday morning or turn off your screens an hour earlier during the highest-mileage weeks. The extra rest that gets you to the start line healthy will be worth it.

RACE STRATEGY

The marathon requires focus and discipline to execute well. By the time you get to the start line, you'll have a goal pace in mind. But during such a long race, you're going to have variables in each mile—hills, bridges, wind, turns, water stations, big crowds, and dicey footing. These factors can slow you down during some miles and allow you to pick up speed during others.

So I suggest a "bubble" for a goal pace instead of a set number. You can have an average that you're aiming for—say, seven or eight minutes per mile. But you should allow yourself to feel satisfied with any miles that are 30 seconds on either side of your goal pace. So shooting for 6:30 to 7:30 for seven-minute miles or 7:30 to 8:30 for eight-minute miles represents a great plan.

For the New York City Marathon, for instance, my fastest mile was 5:28 and my slowest, 6:33—an average of 5:53. Another thing to remember is that in big-city marathons, your GPS watch may not always sync up properly. Turn off your auto lap feature and instead hit the "lap" button with each mile marker. Better yet, run on effort versus using the watch constantly—just the way I recommend practicing in training.

Note: Conditions will also play a role in setting your goal pace on the day. You might have a number in mind based on your training and on cutoffs for events like the Boston Marathon or the Olympic Trials. But if it's a hot, humid day—or a cold, blustery one—you will likely have to shift what you're aiming for in order to have the best race possible (perhaps adjusting your bubble to 6:45 to 7:45, or 7:45 to 8:45, in the previous examples). If you feel good in the final miles, you might be able to speed up to a pace closer to your original goal—but the odds of that happening are much higher if you're realistic about the situation than if you don't make adjustments. (And if you're running on effort as recommended previously, that accounts for the conditions automatically—another reason it's a great idea!)

As with the half marathon, I break down the marathon into segments and take them one at a time, with a specific focus and mantra for each segment. It's critical not to start too fast, so I spend the early miles aiming to relax and settle into a groove. The toughest part for me is always around halfway, when I've been running a long time but still have a significant way to go. That's when I lean heavily on mantras and positive self-talk to stay focused.

- *Start-5K-10K.* Ease into the race, find your breathing rhythm, and stay relaxed and composed. These things are at the forefront of my focus for the first part of the marathon. I think about getting in my first gel and fluids and establishing my position with those around me.

- *10K-15K-20K.* You've found your rhythm; now, it's all about locking into the groove. Try to use minimal mental and physical energy and check off the miles. I focus on my form and running the tangents—the shortest distance around curves and turns. Some races, such as the Chicago Marathon, mark these for you on the roads.

- *20K-25K-30K.* The tipping point of the halfway mark is both exciting and scary. This is the time to utilize the mental tools that you have developed throughout your training. When those thoughts of doubt creep into my head, I push them out and replace them with positive self-talk and personal mantras.

- *30K-35K.* The fatigue is real, but the end is in sight. At this point in the race, when I'm really feeling the grind, I think back to specific workouts and long runs when I pushed through rough patches and finished strong.

- *35K-finish.* Almost there! Keep your mind sharp and engaged in what you're doing. Turnover, form, breathing, and mindset all need to work together to bring it home. I set smaller goals during this time and break down the race into one-mile segments or even shorter, more tangible markers, such as the upcoming turn, the next water table, or even one telephone pole to the next, whatever I need to continue that forward momentum to the finish line.

Finally, a solid nutrition plan is critical to avoid hitting the dreaded "wall" in the later miles. There's more information in chapter 4, on page 50, but every athlete is different—that's why it's so critical to practice your strategy during long runs. But in brief, I recommend the following to athletes:

- One gel, or package of chews, or whatever source of carbohydrate works for you 5 to 15 minutes before the race
- At least 30 grams of carbohydrate per hour—more if you can stomach it—through gels, chews, sports drinks, or other fuel sources
- Twelve to 20 ounces of fluids per hour

As with the half marathon, it's critical to research what fluids will be provided on the course and whether they'll work for you or you need to carry everything on your own. While some marathons do distribute gels at one or more points along the course, they won't be enough to carry you through all 26.2 miles. So you'll want to plan how to tote your own or have friends or family members to help you along the way.

Table 14.1 Marathon Training Plan, 22-Week Schedule

Week	Monday	Tuesday	Wednesday	Thursday	Friday	Saturday	Sunday	Total mileage
1 Stability segment	**Recovery run** 4-7 miles	**Recovery run** 5-8 miles	**Cross-training** 30-60 min	**Recovery run** 5-8 miles	**Recovery run** 4-7 miles	**Long run** 7-10 miles	**Rest day**	25-40
2 Stability segment	**Recovery run** 5-8 miles	**Recovery run** 5-8 miles	**Cross-training** 30-60 min	**Recovery run** 5-8 miles	**Recovery run** 5-8 miles	**Long run** 8-11 miles	**Rest day**	28-43
3 Stability segment	**Recovery run** 5-8 miles	**Recovery run** 6-9 miles	**Cross-training** 30-60 min	**Recovery run** 6-9 miles	**Recovery run** 5-8 miles *Mobility moves: lower leg and feet routine*	**Long run** 9-12 miles	**Rest day**	31-46
4 Stability segment	**Recovery run** 6-9 miles	**Recovery run** 6-9 miles	**Cross-training** 30-60 min	**Recovery run** 6-9 miles	**Recovery run** 6-9 miles *Mobility moves: lower leg and feet routine*	**Long run** 10-13 miles	**Rest day**	34-49
5 Stability segment	**Recovery run** 6-9 miles	**Recovery run with strides** 6-9 miles with 5×20/40s *Resistance band routine*	**Cross-training** 30-60 min	**Recovery run with strides** 6-9 miles with 5×20/40s	**Recovery run** 6-9 miles *Mobility moves: lower leg and feet routine*	**Long run** 11-14 miles	**Rest day**	35-50
6 Stability segment	**Recovery run** 6-9 miles	**Recovery run with hill sprints** 6-9 miles with 5×20 sec hill sprints *Resistance band routine*	**Cross-training** 30-60 min	**Recovery run with hill sprints** 6-9 miles with 5×20 sec hill sprints	**Recovery run** 6-9 miles *Mobility moves: lower leg and feet routine*	**Long run** 12-15 miles	**Rest day**	36-51
7 Stability segment	**Recovery run** 6-9 miles	**Recovery run with strides** 6-9 miles with 5×20/40s *Resistance band routine*	**Cross-training** 30-60 min	**Negative-split run** 6-9 miles	**Recovery run** 6-9 miles *Mobility moves: lower leg and feet routine*	**Long run** 6×30 sec hard on 90 sec easy in the second half Total: 12-15 miles	**Rest day**	36-51

(continued)

Table 14.1 Marathon Training Plan, 22-Week Schedule *(continued)*

Week	Monday	Tuesday	Wednesday	Thursday	Friday	Saturday	Sunday	Total mileage
8 Stability segment	**Recovery run** 6-9 miles	**Recovery run with hill sprints** 6-9 miles with 5×20 sec hill sprints *Resistance band routine*	**Cross-training** 30-60 min	**Tempo run** 4-6 miles at steady state Total: 7-10 miles	**Recovery run** 6-9 miles *Mobility moves: tight hips*	**Long run** 13-16 miles	**Rest day**	38-53
9 Buildup block	**Recovery run** 6-9 miles	**Fartlek** 2 sets of 6-8×30 sec hard on 90 sec easy with 3 min between sets Total: 6-9 miles *Resistance band routine*	**Cross-training** 30-60 min	**Hills** Hill surge 7-10 miles	**Recovery run** 6-9 miles *Mobility moves: tight hips*	**Long run** 6×1 min hard on 3 min easy in the second half Total: 13-16 miles	**Rest day**	38-53
10 Buildup block	**Recovery run** 6-9 miles	**Hills** 8-12×30 sec hill sprints on easy jog down recovery Total: 6-9 miles *Resistance band routine*	**Cross-training** 30-60 min	**Negative-split run** 7-10 miles	**Recovery run** 6-9 miles *Mobility moves: tight hips*	**Long run** 14-17 miles	**Rest day**	39-54
11 Buildup block	**Recovery run** 6-9 miles	**Fartlek** 2×30 sec on 90 sec, 2×1 min on 2 min, 2×2 min on 2 min, 2×1 min on 2 min, 2×30 sec on 90 sec Total: 7-10 miles *Body weight routine*	**Cross-training** 30-60 min	**Hills** Reverse hill surge run Total: 7-10 miles *Core routine*	**Recovery run** 6-9 miles *Mobility moves: tight hips*	**Long run** 5 miles easy, 4-6×1 mile at marathon pace on 400 m jog, easy miles to get in total volume Total: 14-17 miles	**Rest day**	40-55
12 Buildup block	**Recovery run with strides** 6-9 miles with 5×20/40s	**Hills** 4×30 sec hills on 90 sec jog down, 4×1min hills on 2 min jog down, 4×30 sec hills on 90 sec jog down Total: 7-10 miles *Body weight routine*	**Cross-training** 30-60 min	**Alternations** 5-7 mile tempo run alternating between marathon pace and steady state every mile (start and end with marathon-pace mile) Total: 8-11 miles *Core routine*	**Recovery run** 6-9 miles *Mobility moves: tight hips*	**Long run** 15-18 miles	**Rest day**	42-57

Week	Monday	Tuesday	Wednesday	Thursday	Friday	Saturday	Sunday	Total mileage
13 Buildup block	**Recovery run with hill sprints** 6-9 miles with 5×20 sec hill sprints	**Track workout** 3 miles of straights and turns (run the straights hard and jog the turns of the track) Total: 7-10 miles *Body weight routine*	**Cross-training** 30-60 min	**Combo run** 4×1 min hard on 2 min easy, 2-4 miles at steady state, 4×1 min hard on 2 min easy Total: 8-11 miles *Core routine*	**Recovery run** 6-9 miles *Mobility moves: knee pain or stiffness*	**Long run** Progression (start out easy for the first half, then progress the pace the second half as feels right to you) Total: 15-18 miles	Rest day	42-57
14 Buildup block	**Recovery run with strides** 7-10 miles with 5×20/40s	**Hills** 4×1 min hill, 4×45 sec hill, 4×30 sec hill all on easy jog down recovery Total: 7-10 miles *Body weight routine*	**Cross-training** 30-60 min	**Tempo run** 4-6 miles at marathon pace Total: 7-10 miles *Core routine*	**Recovery run** 6-9 miles *Mobility moves: knee pain or stiffness*	**Long run** 16-19 miles	Rest day	43-58
15 Performance phase	**Recovery run with hill sprints** 7-10 miles with 5×20sec hill sprints	**Fartlek** 8-12×1 min hard on 2 min easy Total: 7-10 miles *Body weight routine*	**Cross-training** 30-60 min	**Combo run** 1-2 sets of 1 mile at steady state on 1 min jog, 1 mile at marathon pace on 2 min jog, 1 mile at half marathon pace on 3 min jog Total: 8-11 miles *Core routine*	**Recovery run** 6-9 miles *Mobility moves: knee pain or stiffness*	**Long run** Pick a route that provides a similar elevation profile to your upcoming race course. Run easy but visualize your race Total: 15-19 miles	Rest day	43-59
16 Performance phase	**Recovery run with strides** 7-10 miles with 5×20/40s	**Repeats** 2 sets of 6-8×200 m starting at 10K and working to 1 mile on 100 m jog with 400 m jog between sets Total: 7-10 miles *Body weight routine*	**Cross-training** 30-60 min	**Tempo run** 5-7 miles at marathon pace Total: 8-11 miles *Core routine*	**Recovery run** 7-10 miles *Mobility moves: knee pain or stiffness*	**Long run** 16-20 miles	Rest day	45-61

(continued)

Table 14.1 Marathon Training Plan, 22-Week Schedule *(continued)*

Week	Monday	Tuesday	Wednesday	Thursday	Friday	Saturday	Sunday	Total mileage
17 Performance phase	**Recovery run with hill sprints** 8-11 miles with 5×20 sec hill sprints	**Intervals** 3-4 sets of 4×400 m starting at half-marathon pace and working to 10K on 100 m jog with 400 m jog between sets Total: 8-12 miles *Dumbbell routine*	**Cross-training** 30-60 min	**Hills** Hill surge run 8-11 miles *Dumbbell routine*	**Recovery run** 7-10 miles *Mobility moves: knee pain or stiffness*	**Long run** Miles 8, 10, 12, and 14 at marathon pace with easy miles between (and before and after) Total: 16-20 miles	**Rest day**	47-64
18 Performance phase	**Recovery run with strides** 8-11 miles with 5×20/40s	**Fartlek** 4×1 min, 4×45 sec, 4×30 sec, 4×15 sec all on 90 sec jog Total: 7-10 miles *Dumbbell routine*	**Cross-training** 30-60 min	**Threshold run** 3-5×1 mile at half-marathon pace on 400 m jog Total: 7-10 miles *Dumbbell routine*	**Recovery run** 7-10 miles *Mobility moves: full body mobility*	**Long run** 16-19 miles	**Rest day**	45-60
19 Performance phase	**Recovery run with hill sprints** 8-12 miles with 5×20 sec hill sprints	**Intervals** 6-8×800 m at 10K pace on 400 m jog Total: 9-12 miles *Dumbbell routine*	**Cross-training** 30-60 min	**Alternations** 7-9 mile tempo alternating between marathon pace and steady state every mile (start and end with marathon pace) Total: 9-13 miles *Dumbbell routine*	**Recovery run** 8-11 miles *Mobility moves: full body mobility*	**Long run** 18-22 miles	**Rest day**	52-70
20 Performance phase	**Recovery run** 6-9 miles	**Recovery run with strides** 8-11 miles with 5×20/40s *Dumbbell routine*	**Cross-training** 30-60 min	**Medium-long run** 9-12 miles *Dumbbell routine*	**Recovery run** 6-9 miles *Mobility moves: full body mobility*	**Long run** 2×4-5 miles with first 4-5 at marathon pace, second 4-5 at marathon pace - 10 seconds with 1 mile recovery jog between Total:12-15 miles	**Rest day**	41-56

Week	Monday	Tuesday	Wednesday	Thursday	Friday	Saturday	Sunday	Total mileage
21 Taper time	**Recovery run with hill sprints** 8-11 miles with 5×20 sec hill sprints	**Fartlek** 3×3 min hard, 3×2 min hard, 3×1 min hard all on 2 min recovery Total: 6-9 miles *Dumbbell routine*	**Cross-training** 30-60 min	**Lactate threshold run** 3-5×1 mile at half-marathon pace on 400 m jog Total: 7-10 miles *Dumbbell routine*	**Recovery run** 5-8 miles *Mobility moves: full body mobility*	**Long run** 11-14 miles	**Rest day**	37-52
22 Taper time	**Recovery run with strides** 6-9 miles with 5×20/40s	**Combo run** 2 miles at steady state, 400 m jog, 2×800 m at marathon pace on 400 m jog Total: 7-9 miles *Dumbbell routine*	**Cross-training** 30-60 min	**Fartlek** 2×1 min hard on 2 min easy, 4×30 sec hard on 90 sec easy Total: 5-7 miles	**Rest day** *Mobilty moves: full body mobility*	**Premeet** 3-5 miles with strides	**Marathon** 26.2 miles	47.2-56.2

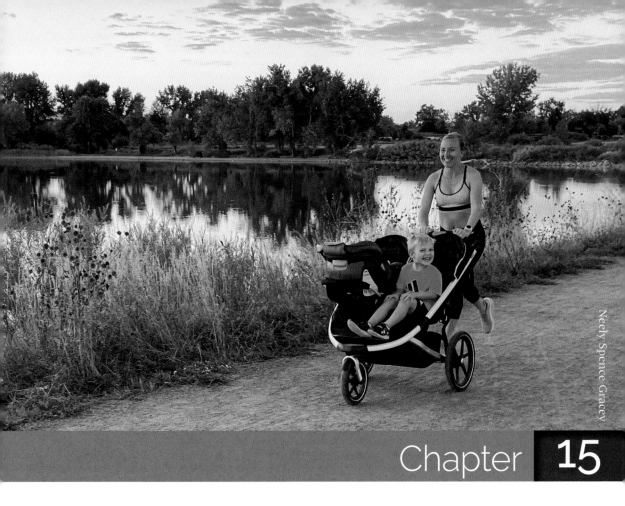

Chapter **15**

Run-Walk Training Plan

From Neely's Log

Breakthrough day: *September 10, 2018*

I'M BACK! Following my six-week postpartum checkup, I headed out for my first run. I ran one minute, walked one minute, 10 times through. Everything felt jiggly and awkward, but it was glorious, nonetheless. My focus is on redeveloping a routine, rebuilding my strength, and—after six weeks of barely opening my training log—beginning to fill it again. I want to run more, but my mantra right now is "patience." I need to take this slowly, recognizing that there will be easy days and hard days but they're all building up to my bigger goals.

GO THE DISTANCE

Whether it's caused by injury, pregnancy, or other life circumstances, you'll most likely end up taking a break from running sometime during your life. Fortunately, running will wait patiently for you until you return. If it's been more than a month or two—and especially if you've been injured or given birth—things will go best if you gradually reacquaint yourself.

You can turn to this plan (table 15.1) anytime you need an on-ramp back after time away. It starts with 15-minute run-walks, for which you'll run, at most, for two minutes at a time. Gradually, you'll progress toward continuous running at a rate that allows your body to adapt and strengthen in a steady progression. Your goal here is not to overload your tissues but to rebuild a routine, gain momentum, and develop consistency.

Each week includes four run-walks or runs, one rest day, and two or three days of cross-training. On the cross-training days, you can use a bike, an elliptical, a stair stepper, a pool for swimming or water running, a hike, or any combination of those options—anything that's lower impact. Feel free to push your heart rate a little higher here with intervals or tempo-like efforts.

Meanwhile, keep your running pace easy; these run-walk days are not designed to be speed workouts. Run comfortably and controlled and know that the walk breaks are there to have you walking before you "need" to. Your goal is to rebuild your body's aerobic system and develop stability and strength in everything from your tendons, ligaments, and bones to your aerobic system, muscles, and mitochondria.

Many high-level athletes are surprised to find returning to running as mentally demanding as harder training, if in a different way. Our natural tendency as athletes is to compare ourselves not just to others but also to previous versions of ourselves, especially at times when we reached our peak fitness. But the key to rebuilding is staying in the moment. Narrow your focus to look only at where you were last week, where you are today, and where you're headed next week.

That's one reason I wrote this plan in minutes instead of mileage. Not only is it logistically challenging to break down run-walks into distance, but going by time also helps you put pace aside and keep the focus on slowly increasing how long you're on your feet. Instead of stressing out about being slow, allow yourself to appreciate the gains you're making in duration.

If you still struggle to slow down or find yourself in your head about pace, you can cover your watch face or turn off the mile splits or even the entire GPS function. Or you can use a simple stopwatch or your phone's stopwatch app to track your time instead.

The plan also includes strength training and mobility work. During those mobility sessions—and in each of your other workouts—pay close attention to the signals your body is sending you. Don't be afraid to repeat weeks if aching, pain, or tightness indicates you're not quite ready to handle an increase in work.

Just to make that even more clear, while I've provided all these details and specifics, laying out this plan week by week as I would any other training program, it's designed to be much more flexible. You should absolutely feel empowered to tailor it to your needs, repeating specific workouts or entire weeks and adding in extra rest days as needed.

There's a lot more about returning to running postpartum in chapter 6, on page 79. But briefly, signs you might need to pause or go more slowly in this situation include new or continued bleeding or a feeling of heaviness in your pelvis, as if your organs are going to fall out if you're not careful. Also, sleep is so hit or miss at this stage. If you're fatigued, you'll often get more benefit from spending an extra hour snoozing than squeezing in a run in the early morning or during baby's nap time.

So again, use this plan as a loose guide only, not a way to judge yourself or set an expectation of what you "should" be doing. If you feel good and want to take the next step forward, great! But if you want or need to stay in a given phase for a while or take a step back, that's far better than moving forward too quickly.

Similar advice holds when you're returning from injury. No training block is going to go exactly as you expect it, building in a straight line from where you are to where you want to be. That's extra true when your body is recovering from a stress such as an injury or pregnancy. It's truly incredible what our tissues can do to repair themselves and even grow stronger and more resilient, but the process can sometimes take more time than we expect or would prefer. Progressing a little more slowly isn't a sign of failure or weakness; at this stage of the game, being mentally tough means being honest with yourself and holding back a bit when necessary. Small forward motion will get you where you want to go, I promise!

Table 15.1 Run-Walk Training Plan, 12-Week Schedule

Week	Monday	Tuesday	Wednesday	Thursday	Friday	Saturday	Sunday	Total Milage
1	**Run-walk** 5×run 1 min/walk 2 min	**Cross-training** 20 min	**Run-walk** 10×run 1 min/walk 1 min *Resistance band routine*	**Rest day**	**Run-walk** 5×run 2 min/walk 2 min	**Cross-training** 20 min *Mobility moves: lower leg and feet routine*	**Rest day**	**Run-walk** 55 min **Cross-training** 40 min
2	**Run-walk** 8×run 2 min/walk 1 min	**Cross-training** 25 min	**Run-walk** 5×run 3 min/walk 2 min *Resistance band routine*	**Rest day**	**Run-walk** 7×run 3 min/walk 1 min	**Cross-training** 25 min *Mobility moves: tight or sore shoulders*	**Rest day**	**Run-walk** 1 hr, 17 min **Cross-training** 50 min
3	**Run-walk** 5×run 4 min/walk 2 min	**Cross-training** 30 min	**Run-walk** 6×run 4 min/walk 1 min *Resistance band routine*	**Rest day**	**Run-walk** 5×run 5 min/walk 2 min	**Cross-training** 30 min *Mobility moves: tight hips*	**Rest day**	**Run-walk** 1 hr, 35 min **Cross-training** 1 hr
4	**Run-walk** 6×run 5 min/walk 1 min	**Cross-training** 30 min	**Run-walk** 5×run 6 min/walk 2 min *Core routine*	**Cross-training** 30 min	**Run-walk** 6×run 6 min/walk 1 min	**Cross-training** 30 min *Mobility moves: tight or sore lower back*	**Rest day**	**Run-walk** 1 hr, 58 min **Cross-training** 1 hr, 30 min
5	**Run-walk** 5×run 7 min/walk 2 min	**Cross-training** 30 min	**Run-walk** 6×run 7 min/walk 1 min *Core routine*	**Cross-training** 35 min	**Run-walk** 4×run 8 min/walk 2 min	**Cross-training** 40 min *Mobility moves: knee pain or stiffness*	**Rest day**	**Run-walk** 2 hr, 13 min **Cross-training** 1 hr, 45 min
6	**Run-walk** 5×run 8 min/walk 1 min	**Cross-training** 35 min	**Run-walk** 5×run 9 min/walk 2 min *Resistance band routine*	**Cross-training** 40 min	**Run-walk** 5×run 9 min/walk 1 min	**Cross-training** 45 min *Mobility moves: full body mobility*	**Rest day**	**Run-walk** 2 hr, 30 min **Cross-training** 2 hr

Week	Monday	Tuesday	Wednesday	Thursday	Friday	Saturday	Sunday	Total Milage
7	**Recovery run** 25 min	**Cross-training** 40 min	**Recovery run** 30 min *Body weight routine*	**Cross-training** 45 min	**Recovery run** 35 min	**Cross-training** 50 min *Select a mobility routine that supports your body*	Rest day	**Running** 1 hr, 30 min **Cross-training** 2 hr, 15 min
8	**Recovery run** 30 min	**Cross-training** 45 min	**Recovery run** 35 min *Body weight routine*	**Cross-training** 50 min	**Recovery run** 40 min	**Cross-training** 55 min *Select a mobility routine that supports your body*	Rest day	**Running** 1 hr, 45 min **Cross-training** 2 hr, 30 min
9	**Recovery run** 35 min	**Cross-training** 50 min	**Recovery run** 40 min *Body weight routine*	**Cross-training** 55 min	**Recovery run** 45 min	**Cross-training** 60 min *Select a mobility routine that supports your body*	Rest day	**Running** 2 hr **Cross-training** 2 hr, 45 min
10	**Recovery run** 40 min	**Cross-training** 60 min	**Recovery run** 45 min *Dumbbell routine*	**Cross-training** 60 min	**Recovery run** 30 min	**Recovery run** 50 min *Select a mobility routine that supports your body*	Rest day	**Running** 2 hr, 45 min **Cross-training** 2 hr
11	**Recovery run** 45 min	**Cross-training** 60 min	**Recovery run** 45 min *Dumbbell routine*	**Cross-training** 60 min	**Recovery run** 30 min	**Recovery run** 55 min *Select a mobility routine that supports your body*	Rest day	**Running** 2 hr, 55 min **Cross-training** 2 hr
12	**Recovery run** 50 min	**Cross-training** 60 min	**Recovery run** 50 min *Dumbbell routine*	**Cross-training** 60 min	**Recovery run** 30 min	**Recovery run** 60 min *Select a mobility routine that supports your body*	Rest day	**Running** 3 hr, 10 min **Cross-training** 2 hr

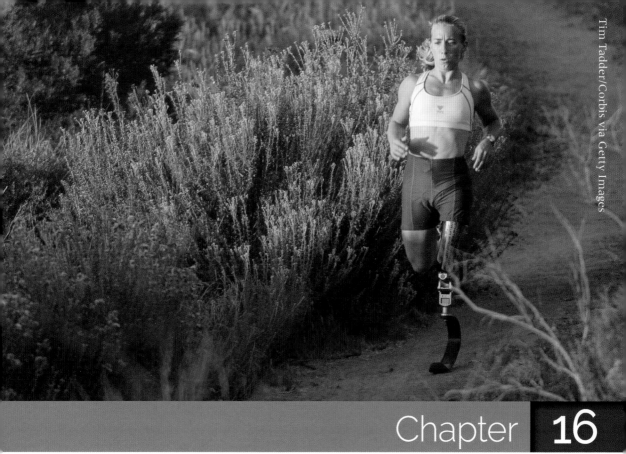

Chapter **16**

Reset for Success

❝ Sometimes forced rest—especially for very driven distance runners—is what we really need to reach the next level, but that only becomes apparent in hindsight. ❞

Becky Wade, elite marathoner, mother, and author of *Run the World*

No matter how diligent you are with goal setting and planning, there are going to be times when unexpected obstacles interfere with your ambitions. Whether it's an illness, injury, or worldwide pandemic, factors beyond your control may require reevaluating your goals and training.

This can feel frustrating, disappointing, infuriating, and even heartbreaking. All those emotions are completely normal and valid; when you go all in on a big goal, you can start to feel an unstoppable drive to achieve it. However, the truth of the matter is that no progression is perfect and the biggest breakthroughs often come after something that feels like a huge setback. Learning how to navigate obstacles and adjust your goals to match reality isn't failure. It's actually a critical step toward success.

WRITE YOUR OWN STORY

My 2016 Boston Marathon breakthrough figures prominently in this book. At this point in my career, it's what I'm best known for and the way I'm most frequently introduced on podcasts or in articles. But there's something you might not know—that it almost didn't happen that way at all.

Originally, my plan had been to debut at the marathon distance during the 2016 Olympic Marathon Trials. At the time, it seemed like a foolproof plan. I was gradually working my way up in distance as I went from a miler in high school to a 5,000-meter runner in college. When I started running road races professionally, I took on the 10K and the half marathon. It seemed the longer the race, the more competitive I was.

That fall of 2015, my half marathon training block was going extremely well. I was really starting to think big things could happen for me in the marathon. And where better to find out than a race that would choose the team representing the United States on the world's biggest athletic stage?

The Philly Rock 'n' Roll Half Marathon—on Halloween of 2015—was both a triumph and a turning point. I ran a personal best of 69:59, making me only the 11th American woman to break the 70-minute mark. But around mile five, I felt a pop in my foot after going around a hairpin curve. After I finished the race, I could barely walk, much less jog my way through a cool-down.

An MRI revealed a stress reaction (a bone injury that occurs before a stress fracture) in my navicular, one of the key bones in the middle of the foot. Healing required a month off, followed by a very slow, easy return to running in December. By the time I came back, I'd have only eight weeks to prepare for the Olympic Trials.

As much as I wanted to make my initial dream come true, it began to seem like a terrible idea to rush into my first-ever marathon—and a high-profile one—on such little preparation. Of course, I was upset and angry, and I felt like my dreams were derailed. I grieved that loss, big-time. But after I took some time to process and consult with the people on my team—my health care providers; my coach then, Steve Magness; and Dillon—we devised a new plan to debut at Boston.

Once I made the mental shift to the new goal, my disappointment dissipated, and my motivation soared. I now had an extra month to prepare for the 26.2-mile challenge. Running my first at Boston quickly felt so right; Patriot's Day 2016 marked exactly 26 years and two days since my dad ran the same race, on the day I was born. A novelist couldn't have dreamed up a better plot, and when I crossed the finish line as first American, it truly felt like both a storybook ending and the beginning to a new, exciting chapter.

What I learned then—and what I hope comes through in these pages—is the balance required for success. Yes, you need big goals to motivate and inspire you, but you also need a smart, rational approach to reach them. Sometimes, success requires pushing forward despite pain and struggle. But just as often, reaching your potential involves backing off or changing strategies to acknowledge shifting circumstances. As I found in Boston, that new path might just be even bigger, better, and more fulfilling than plan A anyway.

FEEL YOUR FEELINGS

While it's true that breakthroughs don't come without setbacks, you can't deny that these bumps in the road hurt. When you have a big dream and a detailed plan to achieve it, it's normal for negative emotions to arise when that plan must be altered.

In addition to injuries (discussed in chapter 8), examples of disruptions that might affect your training and racing plans include the following:

- An illness that means you have to recover and reset, then slowly rebuild
- A move, job change, or other shift in circumstances that means you can't train the way you'd planned (For instance, you get a promotion that involves longer hours, or you become the caregiver for a sick or aging family member.)
- Travel, especially if you don't have control over the timing of business trips or family vacations
- A surprise pregnancy

Before you can even begin to contemplate how to reset and adjust, give yourself a day or two to feel. Recognize that you're upset, disappointed, angry, sad, and mourning what you thought would be, whether that's as short term as a week of workouts or as major as missing a big race or skipping an entire season or year (or two in my case).

Many athletes feel selfish or guilty for having these emotions. This came up for many of my runners during the COVID-19 pandemic, when races were being canceled left and right. Athletes were upset, but in the face of people suffering serious illness, death, and economic struggle, they didn't feel they had a "right" to grieve. This tension can also occur if the thing interfering with your goals is actually a positive one, such as a promotion or a pregnancy.

My view on this—and that of many sport psychology experts—is that acknowledging your sadness actually makes you a more empathetic, caring person. You're passionate about your goals and invested in them. If you weren't upset about losing the chance to reach them, even if that loss is temporary, I'd be concerned.

This acknowledgment—and even a little wallowing—isn't self-indulgent. It's necessary, and it can help you move forward. As we mentioned in chapter 8, according to a study in the *Journal of Applied Sport Psychology*, athletes who discussed their feelings about an injury either in a journal or verbally were more likely to report experiencing growth following their setback (Salim and Wadey 2018). Part of that growth can be a deeper connection to the pain and suffering of others, which can motivate you to help them overcome obstacles even as you pursue your own ambitions.

Personally, I'm a talker—I don't feel like I can move on from disappointment without hashing it out with the people closest to me. However, all individuals have their own way of processing and working through these emotions, be it journaling, meditating, crying, eating a pint or two of ice cream, watching reality television, or some or all of the above. If you're feeling stuck in negative emotions or having trouble figuring out what works for you to process them, a sport psychologist, certified mental performance consultant, or therapist can be a big help.

Another note about mental wellness: as more and more pro athletes have made clear in recent years, mental health is a critical component of peak performance as well as being a whole, happy human being. Conditions such as anxiety, depression, obsessive-compulsive disorder, and post-traumatic stress don't represent weakness; they're legitimate medical illnesses that require support and treatment. Greek Olympian, distance runner, and actress Alexi Pappas explains this beautifully in her memoir *Bravey*: "Your brain is a body part that can get injured like any other, and it can also heal like any other" (Pappas 2021). Tending to your mental health early and often, perhaps by confiding in friends or seeking stress relief, can prevent some psychological setbacks. But in some cases, just as with a hamstring tear or a broken bone, you need professional help to get better.

Physical injuries and other disruptions—and even some generally positive life changes, such as pregnancy and new motherhood—often bring on bouts of mental injuries or mental illness. These can also occur at any other point in the life of a typical runner. Warning signs to watch out for include feeling hopeless or worthless, not finding joy in your training (or anything else that used to bring you pleasure), withdrawing from your friends and family, or thinking about hurting yourself or other people. If you spot any of these signs, seek help from a counselor, psychologist, social worker, or other mental health professional (your primary care doctor can usually refer you if you don't know where to start). And if you're in crisis, you can always call the National Suicide Prevention Lifeline at (800) 273-8255 in the United States or chat live at suicidepreventionlifeline.org.

THEN MOVE FORWARD

Once you've allowed yourself a period of mourning and processing, it's time to get real about your next steps. I find the next important phase to be one of gathering information—tracking down as many details as you can to understand the new reality and time frame you're working with and what your process should look like to set and reach new goals.

If you're dealing with injury or illness, you need a qualified health care team (refer back to chapter 8 about building one). Later in this chapter, we also provide more advice on both shorter- and longer-term health conditions.

Every situation is different, but as I work with athletes on navigating setbacks, I have a few rules of thumb I follow. One general guideline is not to cram missed miles into a single day or week because while you might be tempted to make up for what you've missed, doing so can increase your risk of overtraining and injury. Instead, it's almost always better to simply look forward. Table 16.1 can help guide you on exactly how to forge ahead based on how much time you've missed and how close you are to your goal race.

All this assumes that you're going to have ample time to train and recover on the other side of a temporary setback. I know that's not always the case, and if your lifestyle is altered for a significant period of time, you might want to take the last option and run for maintenance and stress relief until you're in a better place to put more emphasis on your running.

Again, this isn't the same as giving up on your goal; it's merely acknowledging reality and shifting your timeline for achieving it. Many athletes who take this approach often find the base mileage they log during a particularly stressful period pays off in even bigger breakthroughs down the line.

Table 16.1   How to Handle Missed Training

If you miss . . .	Do this . . .
A day or two of training	Just get back on schedule where you are; don't try to make up missed mileage.
More than three days in a row	Ease in with at least one or two easy runs before resuming a training plan as scheduled.
Five runs or more	Ease back in for one to two weeks, starting with easy runs and adjusting your workouts and volume to reduce mileage and intensity.
More than one week	Adjust your expectations for the upcoming month. If you're racing that month, consider altering your time goals or even dropping them altogether and running by feel. If you're two months or more out from a race, however, it won't likely be a setback in the long run—you can keep the same goals for your season.
More than two weeks	Consider shutting down entirely until you're recovered or healed or your circumstances change. Then develop a new plan once you're feeling strong and you've established a new routine.

RUN OR REST?

Most runners are tough enough to persevere even if they're not feeling their best. But when you're under the weather, that's usually not a great idea. Illnesses—even mild ones such as the common cold—deplete your body's recovery resources, meaning that even if you're able to run, you probably won't reap the same benefits from your training. Plus, you'll risk prolonging or worsening your condition, which can have a more serious effect on your plans.

While I'm not a medical professional—and you should always check with your doctor if you have concerns about your health—here's how I approach minor respiratory infections or similar conditions for myself and for my athletes.

- *For colds and other minor respiratory bugs.* Skip workouts and long runs and take easy runs by feel. Skipping a day or two to rest completely may help you recover more quickly and won't negatively affect your long-term goals. But if running relieves pressure in your head or loosens the gunk in your nose, it's OK to go for it. (If you track your heart rate, you might notice it's about 10 beats per minute or so higher than normal.)

- *For fevers.* Rest until your body temperature goes down and stays there. An elevated body temperature means your immune system is working hard to fight off an infection or other disruption. Heating yourself more with exercise may slow this process and even cause you to overheat to a dangerous degree. (Here, your heart rate may be about 20 beats per minute higher than normal—a red flag to rest.)

- *For short-term stomach bugs or flu.* Don't run if you have symptoms such as aches, chills, nausea, vomiting, or diarrhea. Wait until two days after you're able to resume eating and drinking normally; then do only easy runs for a week afterward. It takes time to replenish your fluids, fuel, and energy stores after such serious symptoms. Rushing back into hard running too soon means you'll risk injuries as well as a blow to your confidence because you won't be able to perform the way you think you should.

- *For illnesses that last more than a few days.* Sometimes, the flu can knock you out for more than a day or two—symptoms can linger for five days or longer. If that's the case, track your symptoms and resting heart rate (more about how to do this on page 32). Once you feel better and your resting heart rate is less than 10 beats per minute higher than normal, you can likely start running again, though it's a good idea to check in with your doctor if you have any concerns. Take it slow and steady for at least two weeks before you jump back into a training plan. COVID has some other considerations; see more about that on the next page.

Note: If you're consistently coming down with something during training, you might want to pay extra attention to your immune system. While regular exercise improves your immunity overall, hard training can temporarily boost your susceptibility to illness and infection (Da Silveira et al. 2021).

Shore it up with good overall fueling—paying special attention to postrun recovery nutrition, along with key nutrients such as vitamin D, vitamin C, and zinc—and adequate sleep and recovery time. Also, take all the basic precautions that served us so well during the pandemic, including washing your hands frequently and staying away from others who have symptoms of illness, especially in the hours after a workout, long run, or race.

WHEN SICKNESS GETS SERIOUS

While runners are generally a healthy group, we're not immune from more severe or lingering conditions. For instance, both Dillon and I have chronic Lyme disease, a tick-borne illness that's common, especially in Pennsylvania and other parts of the Northeast, but is still difficult to accurately diagnose. His initial symptoms, which included anxiety, depression, and a racing heartbeat, occurred the year after he graduated from college in 2010. Eventually, he had a panic attack so severe that he took an ambulance to the hospital, sure he was having a heart attack, yet every test they gave him came back normal.

It took more than a year before he found a specialist in Lyme disease who gave him a test that's more sensitive and specific, the IGeneX ImmunoBlot test (Liu et al. 2018). Around the time he was diagnosed, I started having symptoms too. Mine included trouble recovering from hard workouts, allergic reactions to certain foods and skin care products, and similar heart palpitations.

Thanks to Dillon's experience, I was diagnosed more quickly, and I went through four months of antibiotic treatments. For some people, antibiotics resolve the issue entirely. I felt better soon afterward, but the next year, my problems returned. In the fall of 2014, I was trying to train and race, but nothing was coming together. I was 24 and a professional athlete, but I could barely summon the energy to do the dishes or get the mail. After a round of antibiotics, it then took time, support for my immune system, and supplements—including vitamin D, vitamin C, and magnesium, which tend to be low in people with chronic Lyme disease—to restore my health and function.

Off and on through the years, I've had flares. Fortunately, my last time taking antibiotics was 2017. In addition to taking care of my nutrition, the key has been to stay on top of any symptoms—noting things such as unusual soreness and heaviness in my legs, a stronger reaction to alcohol and caffeine, disruptions in my breathing, and increased effort on my runs—and proactively resting, along with getting help from doctors who specifically know how to treat Lyme disease. Frankly, it's just like having a medical team who understands your goals as a runner. There's a list of physicians on the website lymedisease.org if this issue affects you and you need a referral.

Similarly, in the past couple of years, many athletes have also recovered from infections with COVID-19. According to Dr. Megan Roche, who's an elite runner and coach and also has her PhD in epidemiology, we're still learning a lot about this disease, but we know its effects vary widely from person to person. Therefore, she says, recovery can look very different for each runner as well.

"I am helping athletes frame the return to training post-COVID as a process that more closely resembles the return to training after an injury that requires recovery, with the understanding that every athlete is different and that time scales may be longer," she says. "The return to training may not follow a linear timeline: symptoms may come and go over the course of recovery and it's important to pay attention to those symptoms."

She recommends athletes who've had COVID—especially if they weren't vaccinated when they got sick—consider getting a full medical workup afterward to help gauge their individual recovery plan, then err on the side of caution when it comes to getting back into training. Both the inflammation triggered by the disease and the distress caused by its symptoms can challenge athletes' mental health, so she also recommends building a solid support team.

"I've seen athletes struggle with the uncertainty of training and racing post-COVID, not knowing what recovery will look like or what comes ahead," she says. To help, she recommends viewing the process as a day-to-day journey, refraining from judging yourself if you don't meet a specific timeline. Focusing on self-care and treating your body well in other ways may also aid in the process.

In the first year of the pandemic, I coached more than a dozen athletes who were sick with COVID. I personally have seen many athletes feel significantly better by about the six-month mark—and Dr. Roche says she's seen much swifter recoveries in those who have gotten COVID after getting vaccinated, versus those who got the disease when they were unvaccinated. But as she points out, there's much we don't yet know about the long-term effects of COVID. Receiving the COVID vaccine if you haven't already, or trying new drug and treatment therapies, may offer some relief, but most important, she says, may be a shift in mindset.

"It can be normal to ask questions like, 'Will I ever be the same?' much in the same way as can happen after a major injury," she says. "I want all athletes to work on developing a belief-oriented, growth mindset, having faith in the individual recovery process and the science that continues to evolve. The exact path forward may be uncertain, but no matter where the twists and turns lead, it will be an adventure. And at every step of the adventure, you are enough just as you are."

Honestly, this advice applies no matter what type of illness or physical setback you're returning from, be it surgery, pregnancy, or illness. While each circumstance is unique, generally, the runners who do best take a patient, controlled, and disciplined approach to returning to activity. When your body's already under stress, less is more. You're more likely to achieve your goals, and sooner, if you honor your process rather than pushing too hard.

Step by Step: Becky Wade

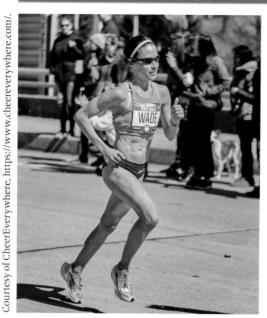

Courtesy of CheerEverywhere, https://www.cheereverywhere.com/.

Most injured athletes fear they'll never be the same after an injury. And elite marathoner Becky Wade—who's also a writer and author of the book *Run the World*—is no exception, she admits. But each time she's been sidelined, she says, she's surprised herself with how strong a comeback she makes.

Take the hip ligament she tore her junior year at Rice University, an injury that required extensive surgery and took her out for nearly two full years. She definitely had moments of struggling during that period, times when she couldn't bear to be around the track and she questioned her future in running. But her first and only time earning all-American honors in cross country happened her first full season back. She also qualified for the Olympic Trials in two events that spring.

"Even though they always suck a lot in the moment, every injury has revealed something about me or my approach that ultimately benefited me," she says. "Every time I choose to persist through dark periods of cross-training, doctor's appointments, and cheering teammates on from the sidelines, it's like I return with a slightly higher ceiling despite the time away."

Exactly how she responds to injuries depends on several factors, including at what point in her training they occur. If the injury occurs near the end of a big marathon build, she'll prepare for the race as best she can, even if that means taking her training to the pool instead. "But if an injury comes on at a time when I'm not super close or locked into anything, I clear my calendar for the immediate future and focus on full healing before I throw myself into getting race ready," she says. "Some people need a race on their schedule to stay motivated, but for me, it tempts me to push too hard or come back too early, and it's better to go one step at a time."

Becky put that into practice in 2020, when not long after the Olympic Marathon Trials, she began feeling soreness in her Achilles tendon. Even though she backed off training when her races were canceled, her pain still worsened. It's been her longest and most frustrating injury, she says, because the timeline is so uncertain. But she's getting through it with the help of an expert physical therapist, diligence with strength and core routines, and a newfound appreciation for what she calls "cross-training proficiency."

"It can take a while to learn how to work hard in the pool and on a bike or machine if you're only used to running and also to get a feel for how running translates to different forms of training," she says. "I'll never like them as much as running, but at least I'm comfortable cross-training and know how to transition back to full running when it's time."

Her biggest advice for coping with the unknowns of recovery is to recall the incredible power of rest. "What helps me any time I'm injured and don't see a way out is to remember that my body is a master at healing," she says. "It's super tempting to throw every possible diagnosis and treatment at it until something seems to move the needle forward, but many times my healing really kicks in when I back off, prioritize rest, and stop stressing so much and forcing a timeline."

FROM BARRIER TO BREAKTHROUGH

Your pathway to greatness probably won't go in the direction you'd planned, but those setbacks make the payoff all the more rewarding.

Barrier

I can't run my goal race, and I just can't get past my feelings of anger and disappointment.

Breakthrough Goals

Choose one or more.

I will do the following:

- Give myself a set period of time—a day to a week—to allow myself those feelings
- Journal about my negative emotions
- Book an appointment with a sport psychologist or certified mental performance consultant for some tips (find options at appliedsportpsych.org)

Barrier

I've come to terms with the fact that my goal isn't possible on the timeline I thought, but I'm not sure what to do next.

Breakthrough Goals

Choose one or more.

I will do the following:

- Gather as much information as possible from doctors, coaches, or any other relevant experts about what a more realistic timeline might be
- Focus on easy running for stress relief, knowing I can train hard again later when the situation changes
- Set a new goal and timeline and allow myself to feel just as excited and motivated to reach that one (If you need ideas and inspiration, go back to chapter 1 on goal setting, page 3, and go through the whole process again based on your new circumstances.)

Barrier

I have a chronic or serious health condition that makes it hard to know when I'll be able to run normally.

Breakthrough Goals

Choose one or more.

I will do the following:

- Seek a health care team who understands both my condition and my running goals
- Write the daily specifics of my treatment plan, such as medication, nutrition, and rest, into my training log so I treat them as part of what keeps me running well
- Accept that my timeline might need to be more generous and flexible but I can still set big goals and work toward them, one day at a time

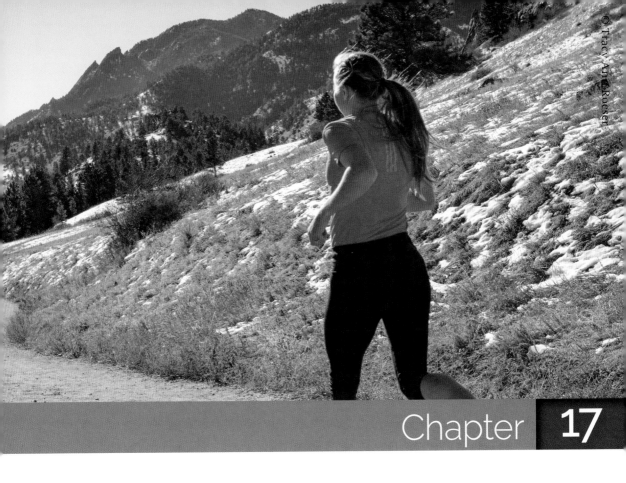
© Tracy Ann Roccer

Chapter | 17

Get It Together

" Some people have little goals, some have big goals, but those who have both are likely to be the most successful. Dream big, my friends, and then start small . . . we never know what's possible unless we try. "

#TrustTheProcess

Neely Agz

By now, you have a solid idea of all the elements that go into a running breakthrough. You've thought through those huge goals that light you up and considered all the small, daily steps that might be required to reach them. It's time to sit down and put together your bigger plan—integrating your big dreams and the breakthrough goals you've set in each chapter into a complete guide to your next big running achievement.

CHART YOUR COURSE

Every runner's story is unique, and within that, each training cycle brings its own set of circumstances. Maybe you're in the position I was before the 2016 Boston Marathon, at a stage in which you'll be able to put more focus and energy than ever into your athletic goals. Or perhaps you're on a journey similar to mine after having Athens—knowing your life is a bit fuller but your competitive fire still burns and aiming to do the most you have in the time available to you.

Each time I start a new training block, I walk through the same basic steps. First, I dream big, thinking about my long-term plans and aspirations. Then I narrow in on a specific race that will cap off this cycle and take me one step closer to where I want to be. I write out my three outcome goals: in the case of the Boston Marathon, running 2:35 or faster, placing in the top 10, and finishing first among Americans. Then I work backward, adding in tune-up races and sketching out the small, daily breakthrough goals that will get me there.

You can think about setting breakthrough goals for each phase of your training cycle—from stability segment to buildup block to performance phase—but I find it often works better to go month by month. The turning of a calendar or planner page marks an easy time to look back at what worked and what didn't and what you want to focus on in the few weeks ahead.

There's no exact ideal number of breakthrough goals you need for each month or phase. I've had as few as 3 and as many as 12. Choose enough to help you bring structure and focus to your training but not so many that you feel overwhelmed.

DRESS REHEARSALS

Part of planning your season is scheduling races along the way. Every runner is a bit different when it comes to racing style. Some people prefer a single big goal race, whereas others would line up every weekend if they could.

Play to your strengths, of course, but in my opinion the best option is a happy medium. If you race too often, you may burn out, not have the time to get in the focused training that is so important, and lack enough recovery time to truly reach your potential. But even though I encourage athletes to select an A race, I don't think it's a great idea to put every egg in that one basket. Racing a few times in your buildup not only gives you other chances to accomplish goals, but it also helps you fine-tune your processes and approach—everything from your clothing and gear to your race-morning mood and routine.

Generally, I recommend racing about once per month, starting in the second or third month of your training block. Mixing up distances is best so you get a wide range of experiences, although the specifics will depend on your goals and circumstances. There's more about how to schedule these in—and adjust your training schedule around them—in chapter 11, on page 153.

Keep in mind that each set of breakthrough goals will build on the prior ones. I find it helps to review how things went with those goals, then for the next month do the following:

- *Fine-tune.* Say you've set an early bedtime but notice that when you get there, you have trouble drifting off. You might add a breakthrough goal to turn off your screens for an hour before and read a book instead.
- *Upgrade.* For instance, if two days of mobility work are going well, add a third!
- *Maintain.* Some breakthrough goals may start to feel more natural, like habits, and require less conscious effort. You can simply leave them as part of your routine and take advantage of the extra bandwidth to add new areas of focus.

Finally, I revisit my outcome goals midway through my training cycle and again right when taper time hits. I look back on the training I've done and make sure my ideas about times and placements are still a good fit—challenging but possible. I derive confidence from revisiting all the hard work I've put in and feel ready to give it my best effort once I get to the start line.

To make all this easier, you can download a set of worksheets on my website, getrunningcoaching.com/breakthrough. There, you'll also find videos of the strength-training routines in this book, additional recipes, and many more tools to help you pull together your breakthrough season.

SEE IT, BE IT

I've been planning this way since high school and college, and I guide my athletes through a similar process. This entire book has been my effort to walk you through it too! But to help you visualize these multitier goals in an even more concrete way, I'm going to take you behind the scenes of a typical client.

Imagine a runner—let's call her Cadence—who's in her early 30s. She has two young children, a full-time job, and a supportive partner. She fell in love with running in high school track and cross country but pursued other goals in college. Once she graduated, she gravitated back toward racing as a source of structure and routine as well as a way to connect with friends.

She trained in groups and ran several marathons, including the Boston Marathon, before marriage and family life took priority. Now, with her kids in school full-time and a flexible work-from-home schedule, she's aiming to get back into her groove and to run a marathon at a pace similar to or faster than what she ran before giving birth. Here's a sample of the way her big dreams and breakthrough goals might align for this training block.

Goal Race: Chicago Marathon, in Early October

Initial thoughts: I've always wanted to run all the World Marathon Majors, and this flat, fast course gives me optimal odds of running my best time. Starting in April, I'll have six months to plan and train. Working backward, this means I'll sign up for a half marathon in August or September as well as some shorter races in the summer.

I can do four or five runs per week, and I'm comfortable maxing out around 55 or 60 miles, plus a day of cross-training. So I plan to follow the marathon training plan on page 175, sticking to middle-mileage options.

While some of my previous running habits will no doubt carry over, my life looks different now. I still have a GPS watch; a few familiar trails and routes near my house; and a brand of gels that's worked for my stomach, though it's been a while since I've tasted one. But given my need for flexibility, I plan to train mostly on my own instead of in a group, coordinating with a few of my friends for long runs when I can.

I also know I need to talk with my husband about why this goal is so important to me and what types of support I need to reach it. The earlier I have conversations about childcare or a little extra help around the house, the better! I also want to take my family on a mini vacation after the race, so travel planning is another early priority.

Outcome Goals

I've run consistently, with breaks for my pregnancies, and have been getting back into racing 5Ks and 10Ks postpartum. Based on those times and knowing that I'll put in the hard work to move up in distance, as I see them now, my goals are as follow:

1. To get close to my previous personal best, 3:26 (After my tune-up races, I'll reevaluate whether I could aim even faster.)
2. To requalify for the Boston Marathon (I need a 3:30 or better.)
3. To reach the starting line healthy and finish knowing I put it all out there

Month One

My main objective is getting into a routine to lay the foundation for good habits that will keep me strong as my mileage increases. My plan is to get up early and knock out a few emails, drop off my kids at school, and run before I officially start my workday. After pregnancy, I know my glutes are weak and my hips get sore, so I need to stay on top of mobility and strength work.

Breakthrough Goals

1. Wear running clothes to drop off kids
2. Turn the lights out by 9:00 p.m.
3. Twice a week, after the kids are in bed, spend 5 to 10 minutes doing hip mobility exercises

Month Two

Now that I'm adding in speedwork, it's a good time to start practicing mental strategies, such as mantras and mini goals (see page 133). I'm in the groove with my mobility work but realize I also need strength and core training to run my best. Also, I'm starting to notice I feel more fatigued at certain times of the month—I'd like to know where I'm at in my cycle and how to manage my hormones.

Breakthrough Goals

1. Create meaningful mantras and try them out on tougher training days (two to start with: "You can do hard things" and "Trust the process")
2. Add two days a week of lifting or core work so I'm doing strength and mobility four days total
3. Download a period app, such as Fitrwoman (see chapter 5, page 60), to start tracking my cycle

Month Three

As my long-run distances continue to increase, I'll fine-tune my nutrition and hydration. As I get into some hill sprints and tempo runs and line up a rust-buster race, I'm also starting to think more about my breathing. I've been incorporating rhythmic breathing while walking and will start to carry these patterns over to my running.

Breakthrough Goals

1. Practice fueling and hydration on every long run and testing some new options
2. Implement a breathing rhythm focus to help me pace myself and stay calm during harder efforts
3. Sign up for and complete a fitness test race (perhaps a 10K or 10-miler)

Month Four

I'm really starting to dial in what works for me when it comes to balancing intense training with parenthood, work, and life. What once felt like a challenge is now the status quo. I'm going to stick to the same basic formula, aiming to minimize distractions and stress as much as I can and reaching out for help when I need it.

Breakthrough Goals

1. Say no to extras I might take on at other times (For instance, maybe I'll hold off on joining that new book club or PTA committee until after the race.)
2. Coordinate long-run schedules with friends so I'm not doing all those miles alone

(continued)

Goal Race *(continued)*

3. Work out a little extra help with kids, cooking, and errands (Maybe the babysitter can throw in some laundry, we get a meal delivery service for one or two days, or my husband can take an extra night of bedtime duty each week.)

Month Five

This is my final big push—the most intense training and the longest long run—when I'm putting all the pieces together. I know there are times when it's going to feel like a grind, but if I focus on recovery and stay committed to all the small steps I've already implemented, I can emerge from the other side healthy and strong.

Breakthrough Goals

1. Keep my recovery runs easy by checking my breathing or heart rate monitor to remind me to slow down when I need to

2. Add in an extra 5 to 10 minutes of mobility work immediately after my hard runs, targeting areas that feel tighter for me

3. Drink at least 100 ounces of fluid every day to stay hydrated and energized for all my big runs

Month Six

It's almost here—the day I've been working so hard for, circled in red on my calendar! The energy I have been putting into training will now shift into resting well, eating well, and preparing my body and mind to perform.

Breakthrough Goals

1. Schedule a prerace massage, which will relieve any lingering tightness and leave my muscles ready to fire at full throttle

2. Review my training logs to check my outcome goals as well as remembering all the hard work I've put in

3. Stay off my feet as much as I can

Joy as a Compass: Megan Roche

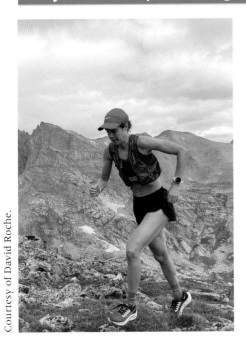

Courtesy of David Roche.

Whether it's on a mountain run or a gravel bike or in a lab, Megan Roche is no stranger to setting big goals—and crushing them.

She is a five-time trail-running national champion, the North American Mountain Running Champion, and a seven-time member of Team USA and has prevailed at distances from 10K to 50 miles. She's a coach who, with her husband David Roche, oversees a thriving community of elite and sub-elite runners called Some Work, All Play (the two also cohost a podcast with the same name and coauthored a book, *The Happy Runner: Love the Process, Get Faster, Run Longer*). And, she's an MD who's earning her PhD in epidemiology while publishing important research on injury in runners, especially women.

With so many skills and talents, Megan has to narrow down the goals and dreams that matter most. To choose, she follows a guiding force, which she calls a joy compass. "As more and more opportunities present themselves, I try to filter decisions through the 'heck yes' or 'heck no' framework—only taking projects on if there's a strong 'heck yes' answer," she says.

Like many top performers, Megan often puts a lot of pressure on herself. So she follows her ambitions in all these avenues but allows herself to be flexible as things unfold. "I find if I hold too tight to goals, they start to become expectations," she says. "So it's most important for me to dream big, without judging myself if goals aren't met or have to be pivoted in new directions."

Even for such a well-rounded, accomplished athlete, big dreams can feel daunting. Setting small, daily steps to reach them keeps her confidence high. These daily process goals also offer her an ongoing progression of clean slates upon which to write her future so she doesn't judge herself when things don't work out exactly as planned. "A single day is just one data point and not a life trajectory," she proclaims.

Through the years, she's coped with plenty of setbacks, including six months when she couldn't run because of a hamstring injury and another several months off of exercise entirely due to heart issues. When that happens, she focuses on expanding her interests outside of running, including science studies, work projects, and creative endeavors. "I've also realized that everyone is still a part of the running community, no matter current or future status with running," she says. "I've enjoyed living vicariously through others, though I also make sure I protect my mental health and energy on days when I feel like I need a break from talking about running."

Coaching, too, helps her keep her perspective and recognize the universality of all parts of the athletic experience. "I've gotten to see that almost all athletes go through similar things—self-doubt, elements of perfectionism, prerace nerves, questioning what matters—and this has helped me extend compassion to myself and empathy to others," she says. In fact, setbacks shouldn't be viewed as failures but as "a side effect of striving and being human. I think if more runners could see how normal this is, it would eliminate a lot of judgment when things get hard and create an even stronger sense of community."

GET RACE READY

Raise your hand if you've been here: For months, your race seems like it'll never arrive. Then, suddenly, it's around the corner, and you can't help but freak out.

My arm is high in the air, and so is that of every athlete I've coached. Prerace jitters are completely normal—again, I take them as a sign you're invested in the outcome. When I start to feel them, I harness this extra adrenaline and put the energy into steps that help me feel organized and in control. Following are four ideas you can consider.

Dial in the Details

By now, you probably have your race website bookmarked; head back to it and read over all the policies and procedures. Make sure you know where and when to pick up your packet, how to get to the starting line, where the water and fuel stations are located, and what postrace events are offered. You'll feel more relaxed once you develop a plan for the flow of the weekend.

Pick a Playlist

Consider the mood you hope to channel on race morning and start assembling a set of tunes that will get you there. Maybe you need upbeat songs to get pumped, or calming music to ease your nerves, or some options for both situations! You can even ask your friends and family for suggestions; that way, you'll wind up with songs full of meaning from those who care about you the most.

Meal Plan

If you're traveling to your race location, scout out the options for local restaurants that serve your prerace meal of choice. Make some calls or book online to have a table ready for you the night before. Go on the early side so you can fuel up, then relax before turning in at a reasonable hour. Also, consider what time you need to get up—I recommend at least three hours before the start of your race—and whether you need to plan for getting coffee or any prerace food you can't bring with you.

Check Conditions

Consult your weather app of choice to start packing for the predicted forecast. Throw in some extras in case things change; I always take a backup pair of shoes, a long-sleeve shirt or jacket, gloves, and a hat. I'd rather be overprepared than caught scrambling. One word of caution: It's easy to let weather concerns send you into an anxiety spiral. Limit these checks to once a week until race week, then daily; once you've checked and adjusted your packing accordingly, you can cross it off your list of worries. We cannot control the weather, but we can be as prepared as possible.

ONE MORE TIME: YOU'VE GOT THIS!

Of course, you likely still have miles to run to reach your goal, but if you've gotten this far, I want to give you a few final words of encouragement for your efforts. You've taken your running and yourself seriously enough to plow through an entire book on how to get the absolute best out of yourself. And if I had to guess, I'd imagine you've been furiously taking notes and bookmarking pages the whole way.

I wholeheartedly believe in you. As I said way back in chapter 1, I can often see athletes' breakthroughs coming, and I know yours is on the way. But I also want you to know you're enough without them. Just by shooting for the stars and planning your path to get there, you've already accomplished so much. I hope you'll take a moment to embrace this beautiful challenge and celebrate your efforts—then get out there and take the next small step toward your biggest, boldest dreams.

References

Chapter 1

Chavez, Chris. 2019. "Gwen Jorgensen Withdraws from 2020 U.S. Olympic Marathon Trials." *Sports Illustrated*. Accessed December 29, 2020. www.si.com/olympics/2019/12/04/gwen-jorgensen-olympics-2020-tokyo-marathon-withdrawal-track-announcement.

Crouse, Lindsay. 2020. "Opinion: She Turned 2020 Misery Into a Breakthrough." *New York Times*, December 26, 2020. www.nytimes.com/2020/12/26/opinion/Sara-Hall-marathon-runner-united-states.html.

Loudin, Amanda. 2021. "How to Set Goals You'll Actually Achieve." *Time*, January 4, 2021. https://time.com/5909923/how-to-set-goals.

Chapter 2

Fleshman, Lauren, and Roisin McGettigan-Dumas. 2014. *Believe Training Journal*. Boulder, CO: VeloPress.

Kuzma, Cindy. 2015. "7 Things We Learned About Marathon Record-Holder Deena Kastor." *ASweatLife*. August 16, 2015. https://asweatlife.com/2015/08/7-things-we-learned-about-marathon-record-holder-deena-kastor.

Nigg, B. M., J. Baltich, S. Hoerzer, and H. Enders. 2015. "Running Shoes and Running Injuries: Mythbusting and a Proposal for Two New Paradigms: 'Preferred Movement Path' and 'Comfort Filter.'" *British Journal of Sports Medicine* 49 (20): 1290-94. https://doi.org/10.1136/bjsports-2015-095054.

Chapter 3

Burfoot, Amby. 2020. "Steve Spence's Best Race, and How He Achieved It." *PodiumRunner*, November 19, 2020. www.podiumrunner.com/training/marathon-training/steve-spences-best-race-and-how-he-achieved-it.

Clarke, Mike J., Cathryn Broderick, Sally Hopewell, Ed Juszczak, and Anne Eisinga. 2016. "Compression Stockings for Preventing Deep Vein Thrombosis in Airline Passengers." *Cochrane Database of Systematic Reviews* 2016 (9). https://doi.org/10.1002/14651858.CD004002.pub3.

Murray, Robert, and W. Larry Kenney. 2016. *Practical Guide to Exercise Physiology*. Champaign, IL: Human Kinetics.

Petrofsky, Jerrold S., Iman Akef Khowailed, Haneul Lee, Lee Berk, Gurinder S. Bains, Siddhesh Akerkar, Jinal Shah, Fuad Al-Dabbak, and Mike S. Laymon. 2015. "Cold vs. Heat After Exercise: Is There a Clear Winner for Muscle Soreness?" *Journal of Strength and Conditioning Research* 29 (11): 3245-52. https://doi.org/10.1519/JSC.0000000000001127.

"Recovery Pace for Runners (With Guest Speaker Steve Spence)." December 16, 2020. Video, 18:45. www.youtube.com/watch?v=UD1RF8cCtuc&t=433s.

Shadgan, Babak, Amir H. Pakravan, Alison Hoens, and W. Darlene Reid. 2018. "Contrast Baths, Intramuscular Hemodynamics, and Oxygenation as Monitored by Near-Infrared Spectroscopy." *Journal of Athletic Training* 53 (8): 782-87. https://doi.org/10.4085/1062-6050-127-17.

Shechter, Ari, Elijah Wookhyun Kim, Marie-Pierre St-Onge, and Andrew J. Westwood. 2018. "Blocking Nocturnal Blue Light for Insomnia: A Randomized Controlled Trial." *Journal of Psychiatric Research* 96 (January): 196-202. https://doi.org/10.1016/j.jpsychires.2017.10.015.

Spence, Steve. 2011. "How Steve Spence Earned Bronze in 1991." *Runner's World*, June 1, 2011. www.runnersworld.com/advanced/a20808250/how-steve-spence-earned-bronze-in-1991.

Stulberg, Brad, and Steve Magness. 2017. *Peak Performance: Elevate Your Game, Avoid Burnout, and Thrive with the New Science of Success*. New York: Rodale.

Vitale, Kenneth C., Robert Owens, Susan R. Hopkins, and Atul Malhotra. 2019. "Sleep Hygiene for Optimizing Recovery in Athletes: Review and Recommendations." *International Journal of Sports Medicine* 40 (8): 535-43. https://doi.org/10.1055/a-0905-3103.

Watson, Andrew M. 2017. "Sleep and Athletic Performance." *Current Sports Medicine Reports* 16 (6): 413-18. https://doi.org/10.1249/JSR.0000000000000418.

Chapter 4

Daley, Cynthia A., Amber Abbott, Patrick S. Doyle, Glenn A. Nader, and Stephanie Larson. 2010. "A Review of Fatty Acid Profiles and Antioxidant Content in Grass-Fed and Grain-Fed Beef." *Nutrition Journal* 9 (1): 10. https://doi.org/10.1186/1475-2891-9-10.

Ellis, E. 2020. "Caffeine and Exercise." *Eat Right*. February 17, 2020. www.eatright.org/fitness/sports-and-performance/fueling-your-workout/caffeine-and-exercise.

Flanagan, Shalane, and Elyse Kopecky. 2016. *Run Fast. Eat Slow: Nourishing Recipes for Athletes*. Emmaus, PA: Rodale.

Flanagan, Shalane, and Elyse Kopecky. 2018. *Run Fast. Cook Fast. Eat Slow. Quick-Fix Recipes for Hangry Athletes*. New York: Rodale.

Gao, Qi, Tingyan Kou, Bin Zhuang, Yangyang Ren, Xue Dong, and Qiuzhen Wang. 2018. "The Association between Vitamin D Deficiency and Sleep Disorders: A Systematic Review and Meta-Analysis." *Nutrients* 10 (10). https://doi.org/10.3390/nu10101395.

Gordon, Barbara A. 2019. "Choose Healthy Fats." Academy of Nutrition and Dietetics. August 6, 2019. www.eatright.org/food/nutrition/dietary-guidelines-and-myplate/choose-healthy-fats.

Guest, Nanci S., Trisha A. VanDusseldorp, Michael T. Nelson, Jozo Grgic, Brad J. Schoenfeld, Nathaniel D. M. Jenkins, Shawn M. Arent, et al. 2021. "International Society of Sports Nutrition Position Stand: Caffeine and Exercise Performance." *Journal of the International Society of Sports Nutrition* 18 (1): 1. https://doi.org/10.1186/s12970-020-00383-4.

Klemm, Sarah. "What Are B-Vitamins?" 2021. *Eat Right*. January 15, 2021. www.eatright.org/food/vitamins-and-supplements/types-of-vitamins-and-nutrients/what-are-b-vitamins-and-folate.

Kong, Peiling, and Lynne M. Harris. 2015. "The Sporting Body: Body Image and Eating Disorder Symptomatology among Female Athletes from Leanness Focused and Nonleanness Focused Sports." *Journal of Psychology* 149 (2): 141-60. https://doi.org/10.1080/00223980.2013.846291.

Melin, Anna K., Ida A. Heikura, Adam Tenforde, and Margo Mountjoy. 2019. "Energy Availability in Athletics: Health, Performance, and Physique." *International Journal of Sport Nutrition and Exercise Metabolism* 29 (2): 152-64. https://doi.org/10.1123/ijsnem.2018-0201.

National Eating Disorders Association (NEDA). 2021. "Warning Signs and Symptoms." Accessed August 17, 2021. www.nationaleatingdisorders.org/warning-signs-and-symptoms.

National Institutes of Health, Office of Dietary Supplements. n.d.a. "Iron." Accessed March 22, 2021. https://ods.od.nih.gov/factsheets/Iron-Consumer.

National Institutes of Health, Office of Dietary Supplements. n.d.b. "Magnesium." Accessed March 22, 2021. https://ods.od.nih.gov/factsheets/Magnesium-Consumer.

Roche, David. 2020. "Fasted Training May Have Long-Term Risks, Especially for Female Athletes." *Trail Runner Magazine.* January 6, 2020. https://trailrunnermag.com/training/fasted-training-may-have-long-term-risks-especially-for-female-athletes.html.

Schoenfeld, Brad Jon, and Alan Albert Aragon. 2018. "How Much Protein Can the Body Use in a Single Meal for Muscle-Building? Implications for Daily Protein Distribution." *Journal of the International Society of Sports Nutrition* 15 (February 27). https://doi.org/10.1186/s12970-018-0215-1.

Thomas, D. Travis, Kelly Anne Erdman, and Louise M. Burke. 2016. "Position of the Academy of Nutrition and Dietetics, Dietitians of Canada, and the American College of Sports Medicine: Nutrition and Athletic Performance." *Journal of the Academy of Nutrition and Dietetics* 116 (3): 501-28. https://doi.org/10.1016/j.jand.2015.12.006.

Vitale, Kenneth, and Andrew Getzin. 2019. "Nutrition and Supplement Update for the Endurance Athlete: Review and Recommendations." *Nutrients* 11 (6). https://doi.org/10.3390/nu11061289.

Chapter 5

BBC Sport. 2015. "Paula Radcliffe: Sport Has Not Learned about Periods." January 22, 2015. www.bbc.co.uk/sport/athletics/30927245.

Centers for Disease Control and Prevention. 2020. "Contraception: Birth Control Methods." Last modified August 13, 2020. www.cdc.gov/reproductivehealth/contraception/index.htm.

Cleveland Clinic. n.d. "Toxic Shock Syndrome." Accessed July 11, 2021. https://my.clevelandclinic.org/health/diseases/15437-toxic-shock-syndrome.

Dean, Teresa M., Leigh Perreault, Robert S. Mazzeo, and Tracy J. Horton. 2003. "No Effect of Menstrual Cycle Phase on Lactate Threshold." *Journal of Applied Physiology* 95 (6): 2537-43. https://doi.org/10.1152/japplphysiol.00672.2003.

Healthline. n.d. "Can Seed Cycling Balance Hormones and Ease Menopause Symptoms?" Accessed July 18, 2019. www.healthline.com/nutrition/seed-cycling.

Krebs, Paul A., Christopher R. Dennison, Lisa Kellar, and Jeff Lucas. 2019. "Gender Differences in Eating Disorder Risk among NCAA Division I Cross Country and Track Student-Athletes." *Journal of Sports Medicine* 2019 (February): e5035871. https://doi.org/10.1155/2019/5035871.

Kuzma, Cindy. 2015a. "Solutions for Runners with Serious Periods." *Runner's World.* September 30, 2015. www.runnersworld.com/women/a20854065/solutions-for-runners-with-serious-periods.

Kuzma, Cindy. 2015b. "What Runners Need to Know about Menstrual Cups." *Runner's World.* September 9, 2015. www.runnersworld.com/women/a20852736/what-runners-need-to-know-about-menstrual-cups.

Kuzma, Cindy. 2020. "The Answers to Every Question You've Ever Had about Menopause and Running." *Runner's World.* October 1, 2020. www.runnersworld.com/women/a20856097/menopause-and-running-what-you-need-to-know.

Kuzma, Cindy. 2021. "Inside Molly Seidel's Bronze Medal Marathon Run in Tokyo." *Runner's World.* August 9, 2021. www.runnersworld.com/runners-stories/a37253992/molly-seidel-olympics-marathon-bronze.

Martin, Dan, Kate Timmins, Charlotte Cowie, Jon Alty, Ritan Mehta, Alicia Tang, and Ian Varley. 2021. "Injury Incidence across the Menstrual Cycle in International Footballers." *Frontiers in Sports and Active Living* 2021 (March 1). https://doi.org/10.3389/fspor.2021.616999.

Mayo Clinic. 2021a. "Estrogen and Progestin Oral Contraceptives (Oral Route)." Last modified February 1, 2021. www.mayoclinic.org/drugs-supplements/estrogen-and-progestin-oral-contraceptives-oral-route/side-effects/drg-20069422.

Mayo Clinic. 2021b. "Perimenopause." Last modified August 7, 2021. www.mayoclinic.org/diseases-conditions/perimenopause/symptoms-causes/syc-20354666.

North American Menopause Society. n.d. "Menopause 101: A Primer for the Perimenopausal." Accessed August 16, 2021. www.menopause.org/for-women/menopauseflashes/menopause-symptoms-and-treatments/menopause-101-a-primer-for-the-perimenopausal.

Office on Women's Health. n.d. "Your Menstrual Cycle." Last modified March 16, 2018. www.womenshealth.gov/menstrual-cycle/your-menstrual-cycle.

Rael, Beatriz, Víctor M. Alfaro-Magallanes, Nuria Romero-Parra, Eliane A. Castro, Rocío Cupeiro, Xanne A. K. Janse de Jonge, Erica A. Wehrwein, and Ana B. Peinado. 2021. "Menstrual Cycle Phases Influence on Cardiorespiratory Response to Exercise in Endurance-Trained Females." *International Journal of Environmental Research and Public Health* 18 (3). https://doi.org/10.3390/ijerph18030860.

Sims, Stacy T., and Selene Yeager. 2016. *ROAR: How to Match Your Food and Fitness to Your Unique Female Physiology for Optimum Performance, Great Health, and a Strong, Lean Body for Life.* Emmaus, PA: Rodale Books.

Singhal, Vibha, Kathryn E. Ackerman, Amita Bose, Landy Paola Torre Flores, Hang Lee, and Madhusmita Misra. 2019. "Impact of Route of Estrogen Administration on Bone Turnover Markers in Oligoamenorrheic Athletes and Its Mediators." *Journal of Clinical Endocrinology & Metabolism* 104 (5): 1449-58. https://doi.org/10.1210/jc.2018-02143.

Society for Endocrinology. 2018. "Melatonin: You and Your Hormones from the Society for Endocrinology." www.yourhormones.info/hormones/melatonin.

Stojanovska, Lily, Vasso Apostolopoulos, Remco Polman, and Erika Borkoles. 2014. "To Exercise, or, Not to Exercise, during Menopause and Beyond." *Maturitas* 77 (4): 318-23. https://doi.org/10.1016/j.maturitas.2014.01.006.

Yan, Hui, Wangbao Yang, Fenghua Zhou, Xiaopeng Li, Quan Pan, Zheng Shen, Guichun Han, et al. 2019. "Estrogen Improves Insulin Sensitivity and Suppresses Gluconeogenesis via the Transcription Factor Foxo1." *Diabetes* 68 (2): 291-304. https://doi.org/10.2337/db18-0638.

Chapter 6

ACOG Committee on Obstetric Practice. 2018. "ACOG Committee Opinion No. 756: Optimizing Support for Breastfeeding as Part of Obstetric Practice." *Obstetrics and Gynecology* 132 (4): e187-96. https://doi.org/10.1097/AOG.0000000000002890.

ACOG Committee on Obstetric Practice. 2020. "ACOG Committee Opinion, Number 804: Physical Activity and Exercise During Pregnancy and the Postpartum Period." *Obstetrics and Gynecology* 135 (4): e178-88. https://doi.org/10.1097/AOG.0000000000003772.

Bø, Kari, Raul Artal, Ruben Barakat, Wendy J. Brown, Gregory A. L. Davies, Michael Dooley, Kelly R. Evenson, et al. 2017. "Exercise and Pregnancy in Recreational and Elite Athletes: 2016/17 Evidence Summary from the IOC Expert Group Meeting, Lausanne. Part 3-Exercise in the Postpartum Period." *British Journal of Sports Medicine* 51 (21): 1516-25. https://doi.org/10.1136/bjsports-2017-097964.

Davenport, Margie H., Amariah J. Kathol, Michelle F. Mottola, Rachel J. Skow, Victoria L. Meah, Veronica J. Poitras, Alejandra Jaramillo Garcia, et al. 2019. "Prenatal Exercise Is Not Associated with Fetal Mortality: A Systematic Review and Meta-Analysis." *British Journal of Sports Medicine* 53 (2): 108-15. https://doi.org/10.1136/bjsports-2018-099773.

Goom, Tom, Grainne Donnelly, and Emma Brockwell. 2019. "Returning to Running Postnatal: -Guidelines for Medical, Health and Fitness Professionals Managing This Population." *Absolute Physio*. March 2019. www.absolute.physio/wp-content/uploads/2019/09/returning-to-running-postnatal-guidelines.pdf.

Healthline. n.d. "Symptoms of Severe Dehydration During Pregnancy." Modified March 3, 2016. www.healthline.com/health/pregnancy/dehydration.

Hew-Butler, T., K. J. Stuempfle, and M. D. Hoffman. 2013. "Bone: An Acute Buffer of Plasma Sodium During Exhaustive Exercise?" *Hormone and Metabolic Research* 45 (10): 697-700. https://doi.org/10.1055/s-0033-1347263.

Johnston, Margreete, Susan Landers, Larry Noble, Kinga Szucs, and Laura Viehmann. 2012. "Breastfeeding and the Use of Human Milk." *Pediatrics* 129 (3): e827-41. https://doi.org/10.1542/peds.2011-3552.

Kuhrt, Katy, Mark Harmon, Natasha L. Hezelgrave, Paul T. Seed, and Andrew H. Shennan. 2018. "Is Recreational Running Associated with Earlier Delivery and Lower Birth Weight in Women Who Continue to Run during Pregnancy? An International Retrospective Cohort Study of Running Habits of 1293 Female Runners during Pregnancy." *BMJ Open Sport & Exercise Medicine* 4 (1): e000296. https://doi.org/10.1136/bmjsem-2017-000296.

Meah, Victoria L., Gregory A. Davies, and Margie H. Davenport. 2020. "Why Can't I Exercise during Pregnancy? Time to Revisit Medical 'Absolute' and 'Relative' Contraindications: Systematic Review of Evidence of Harm and a Call to Action." *British Journal of Sports Medicine* 54 (23): 1395-404. https://doi.org/10.1136/bjsports-2020-102042.

Mottola, Michelle F., Margie H. Davenport, Stephanie-May Ruchat, Gregory A. Davies, Veronica J. Poitras, Casey E. Gray, Alejandra Jaramillo Garcia, et al. 2018. "2019 Canadian Guideline for Physical Activity throughout Pregnancy." *British Journal of Sports Medicine* 52 (21): 1339-46. https://doi.org/10.1136/bjsports-2018-100056.

Salari, Pooneh, and Mohammad Abdollahi. 2014. "The Influence of Pregnancy and Lactation on Maternal Bone Health: A Systematic Review." *Journal of Family & Reproductive Health* 8 (4): 135-48.

Chapter 7

Alexander, James L. N., Christian J. Barton, and Richard W. Willy. 2020. "Infographic. Running Myth: Strength Training Should Be High Repetition Low Load to Improve Running Performance." *British Journal of Sports Medicine* 54 (13): 813-14. https://doi.org/10.1136/bjsports-2019-101168.

Dicharry, Jay. 2017. *Running Rewired: Reinvent Your Run for Stability, Strength and Speed*. Boulder, CO: VeloPress.

Hong, A. Ram, and Sang Wan Kim. 2018. "Effects of Resistance Exercise on Bone Health." *Endocrinology and Metabolism* 33 (4): 435-44. https://doi.org/10.3803/EnM.2018.33.4.435.

Lauersen, Jeppe Bo, Ditte Marie Bertelsen, and Lars Bo Andersen. 2014. "The Effectiveness of Exercise Interventions to Prevent Sports Injuries: A Systematic Review and Meta-Analysis of Randomised Controlled Trials." *British Journal of Sports Medicine* 48 (11): 871-77. https://doi.org/10.1136/bjsports-2013-092538.

Vechetti, Ivan J., Bailey D. Peck, Yuan Wen, R. Grace Walton, Taylor R. Valentino, Alexander P. Alimov, Cory M. Dungan, et al. 2021. "Mechanical Overload-Induced Muscle-Derived Extracellular Vesicles Promote Adipose Tissue Lipolysis." *The FASEB Journal* 35 (6): e21644. https://doi.org/10.1096/fj.202100242R.

Chapter 8

Dallinga, Joan, Rogier Van Rijn, Janine Stubbe, and Marije Deutekom. 2019. "Injury Incidence and Risk Factors: A Cohort Study of 706 8-Km or 16-Km Recreational Runners." *BMJ Open Sport & Exercise Medicine* 5 (1): e000489. https://doi.org/10.1136/bmjsem-2018-000489.

Salim, Jade, and Ross Wadey. 2018. "Can Emotional Disclosure Promote Sport Injury-Related Growth?" *Journal of Applied Sport Psychology* 30 (4): 367-87. https://doi.org/10.1080/10413200.2017.1417338.

Singh, Harnoor, and David E. Conroy. 2017. "Systematic Review of Stress-Related Injury Vulnerability in Athletic and Occupational Contexts." *Psychology of Sport and Exercise* 33 (November 1): 37-44. https://doi.org/10.1016/j.psychsport.2017.08.001.

Van Poppel, Dennis, Gwendolijne G. M. Scholten-Peeters, Marienke van Middelkoop, Bart W. Koes, and Arianne P. Verhagen. 2018. "Risk Models for Lower Extremity Injuries among Short- and Long-Distance Runners: A Prospective Cohort Study." *Musculoskeletal Science and Practice* 36 (August): 48-53. https://doi.org/10.1016/j.msksp.2018.04.007.

Watson, Nathaniel F., M. Safwan Badr, Gregory Belenky, Donald L. Bliwise, Orfeu M. Buxton, Daniel Buysse, David F. Dinges, et al. 2015. "Recommended Amount of Sleep for a Healthy Adult: A Joint Consensus Statement of the American Academy of Sleep Medicine and Sleep Research Society." *Sleep* 38 (6): 843-44. https://doi.org/10.5665/sleep.4716.

Chapter 9

Castaldelli-Maia, João Mauricio, João Guilherme de Mello e Gallinaro, Rodrigo Scialfa Falcão, Vincent Gouttebarge, Mary E. Hitchcock, Brian Hainline, Claudia L. Reardon, et al. 2019. "Mental Health Symptoms and Disorders in Elite Athletes: A Systematic Review on Cultural Influencers and Barriers to Athletes Seeking Treatment." *British Journal of Sports Medicine* 53 (11): 707-21. https://doi.org/10.1136/bjsports-2019-100710.

Hardy, James, Aled V. Thomas, and Anthony W. Blanchfield. 2019. "To Me, to You: How You Say Things Matters for Endurance Performance." *Journal of Sports Sciences* 37 (18): 2122-30. https://doi.org/10.1080/02640414.2019.1622240.

Kuzma, Cindy, and Carrie Jackson Cheadle. 2019. *Rebound: Train Your Mind to Bounce Back Stronger from Sports Injuries.* New York: Bloomsbury.

Walter, Nadja, Lucie Nikoleizig, and Dorothee Alfermann. 2019. "Effects of Self-Talk Training on Competitive Anxiety, Self-Efficacy, Volitional Skills, and Performance: An Intervention Study with Junior Sub-Elite Athletes." *Sports* 7 (6). https://doi.org/10.3390/sports7060148.

Chapter 10

Coates, Budd, and Claire Kowalchik. 2013. *Runner's World Running on Air: The Revolutionary Way to Run Better by Breathing Smarter.* Emmaus, PA: Rodale Books.

Daniels, Jack. 2021. *Daniels' Running Formula.* 4th ed. Champaign, IL: Human Kinetics.

El Helou, Nour, Muriel Tafflet, Geoffroy Berthelot, Julien Tolaini, Andy Marc, Marion Guillaume, Christophe Hausswirth, et al. 2012. "Impact of Environmental Parameters on Marathon Running Performance." *PLOS ONE* 7 (5). https://doi.org/10.1371/journal.pone.0037407.

Morgan, Christine Martin, and Heather K. Vincent. 2017. "Manipulating Cadence for Gait Re-Training in Runners." *Current Sports Medicine Reports* 16 (6): 381. https://doi.org/10.1249/JSR.0000000000000414.

Radak, Zsolt, Zhongfu Zhao, Erika Koltai, Hideki Ohno, and Mustafa Atalay. 2013. "Oxygen Consumption and Usage During Physical Exercise: The Balance Between Oxidative Stress and ROS-Dependent Adaptive Signaling." *Antioxidants & Redox Signaling* 18 (10): 1208-46. https://doi.org/10.1089/ars.2011.4498.

Russo, Marc A., Danielle M. Santarelli, and Dean O'Rourke. 2017. "The Physiological Effects of Slow Breathing in the Healthy Human." *Breathe* 13 (4): 298-309. https://doi.org/10.1183/20734735.009817.

Schubert, Amy G., Jenny Kempf, and Bryan C. Heiderscheit. 2014. "Influence of Stride Frequency and Length on Running Mechanics: A Systematic Review." *Sports Health: A Multidisciplinary Approach* 6 (3): 210-17. https://doi.org/10.1177/1941738113508544.

Chapter 11

Daniels, Jack. *Daniels' Running Formula.* 2021. 3rd ed. Champaign, IL: Human Kinetics.

Chapter 13

Andersen, Jens Jakob. 2021. "The State of Running 2019." *RunRepeat.* September 21, 2021. https://runrepeat.com/state-of-running.

Chapter 16

Da Silveira, Matheus Pelinski, Kimberly Kamila da Silva Fagundes, Matheus Ribeiro Bizuti, Édina Starck, Renata Calciolari Rossi, and Débora Tavares de Resende e Silva. 2021. "Physical Exercise as a Tool to Help the Immune System against COVID-19: An Integrative Review of the Current Literature." *Clinical and Experimental Medicine* 21 (1): 15-28. https://doi.org/10.1007/s10238-020-00650-3.

Liu, Song, Iris Du Cruz, Catherine Calalo Ramos, Paula Taleon, Ranjan Ramasamy, and Jyotsna Shah. 2018. "Pilot Study of Immunoblots with Recombinant *Borrelia Burgdorferi* Antigens for Laboratory Diagnosis of Lyme Disease." *Healthcare (Basel)* 6 (3). https://doi.org/10.3390/healthcare6030099.

Pappas, Alexi. 2021. *Bravey: Chasing Dreams, Befriending Pain, and Other Big Ideas.* New York: Dial Press.

Salim, Jade, and Ross Wadey. 2018. "Can Emotional Disclosure Promote Sport Injury-Related Growth?" *Journal of Applied Sport Psychology* 30 (4): 367-87. https://doi.org/10.1080/10413200.2017.1417338.

Index

About the Authors

Neely Spence Gracey began running in eight grade and quickly saw success, which deepened her motivation to pursue big goals. At the high school level she won four Pennsylvania state championships. Upon graduation, she attended Shippensburg University (SU) and became an eight-time Division II national champion. During Neely's

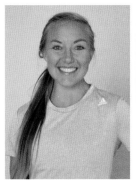
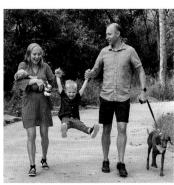

Family photo courtesy of Jill Hampson.

time at SU, she studied human communication with a coaching minor because she knew she wanted to become a pro athlete and start coaching other runners toward their goals.

In 2012, she signed her first pro contract and married her husband Dillon, and in 2013 Get Running Coaching was born. The business has continued to grow, as has Neely's family, with the addition of sons Athens in 2018 and Rome in 2021. She's worked with hundreds of runners all over the world to help them achieve their breakthroughs, from the mile to the marathon. On the roads, she's a three-time Olympic Trials qualifier, was the top American at the 2016 Boston Marathon, and is the 11th American female ever to break 70 minutes in the half marathon. Her personal records are 4:36 for the mile, 15:25 for the 5K, 32:16 for the 10K, 1:09 for the half marathon, and 2:34 for the marathon. She looks forward to her next breakthrough season and has her sights set on qualifying for her fourth Olympic Trials in 2024. The running community inspires her to keep working toward her goals as an athlete, coach, and mother.

Cindy Kuzma is a freelance writer, author, and podcaster; a regular contributor to Runner's World, Women's Running, and a wide variety of other sports, fitness, and health publications; and the coauthor of Rebound: Train Your Mind to Bounce Back Stronger From Sports Injuries. Cindy specializes in covering injury prevention and recovery, everyday athletes who accomplish extraordinary things, and the active community in her beloved Chicago, where winter forges deep bonds between those athletes brave enough to train through it. She has run 22 marathons—including seven in Boston—and she never gets tired of plotting her next breakthrough.

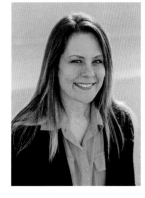

Courtesy of Cindy Kuzma. Photographer: James Wirth.

You read the book—now complete the companion CE exam to earn continuing education credit!

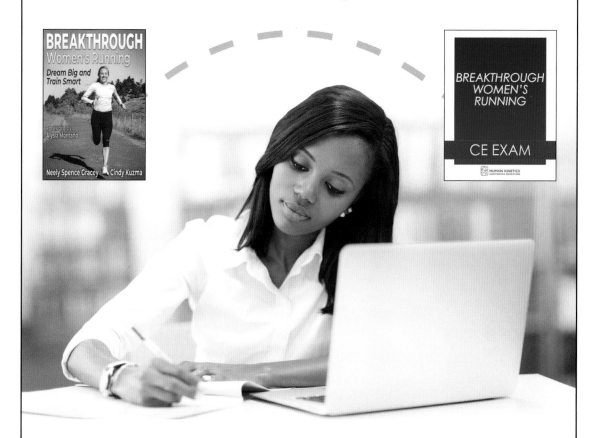

Find and purchase the companion CE exam here:
US.HumanKinetics.com/collections/CE-Exam
Canada.HumanKinetics.com/collections/CE-Exam

50% off the companion CE exam with this code

BWR2023

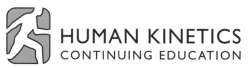

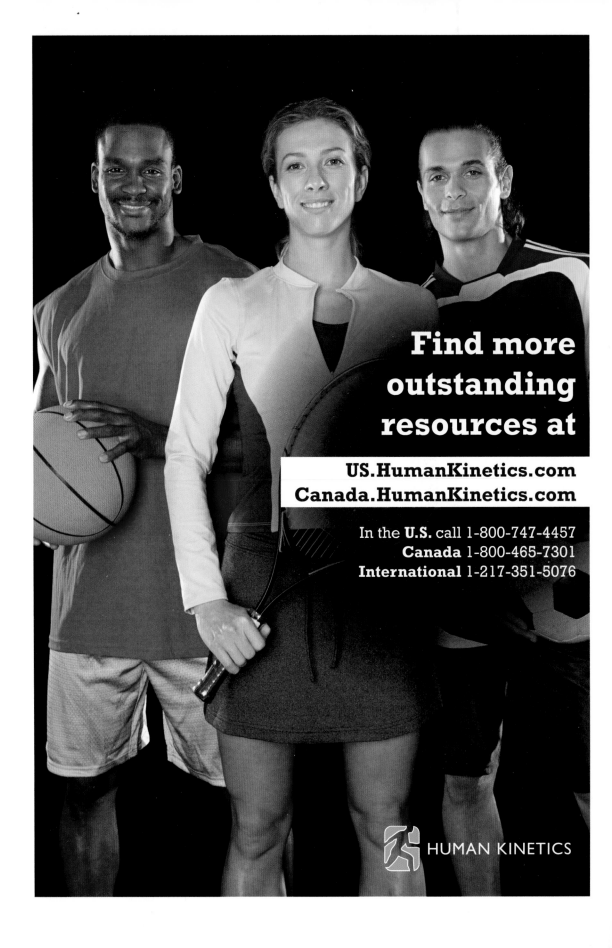